Organoid Bioengineering - Advances, Applications and Challenges

Edited by Manash K. Paul

Published in London, United Kingdom

Organoid Bioengineering - Advances, Applications and Challenges
http://dx.doi.org/10.5772/intechopen.100342
Edited by Manash K. Paul

Contributors
Zi-Bing Jin, Jing Yuan, Haiwei Xu, Jing Gong, Minghui Li, Jun Yang, Jiahui Kang, Xiao Liu, Allen Thayakumar Basanthakumar, Janitha Chandrasekhar-Darlybai, Jyothsna Ganesh, Andrey Popatanasov, Manash K. Paul, Anubhab Mukherjee, Aprajita Sinha, Maheshree Maibam, Bharti Bisht

First published in London, United Kingdom, 2022 by IntechOpen
IntechOpen is the global imprint of INTECHOPEN LIMITED, registered in England and Wales, registration number: 11086078, 5 Princes Gate Court, London, SW7 2QJ, United Kingdom

British Library Cataloguing-in-Publication Data
A catalogue record for this book is available from the British Library

Additional hard and PDF copies can be obtained from orders@intechopen.com

Organoid Bioengineering - Advances, Applications and Challenges
Edited by Manash K. Paul
p. cm.

This title is part of the Biomedical Engineering Book Series, Volume 13
Topic: Biotechnology - Biosensors, Biomaterials and Tissue Engineering
Series Editor: Robert Koprowski
Topic Editor: Luis Villarreal-Gómez

Print ISBN 978-1-80355-768-7
Online ISBN 978-1-80355-769-4
eBook (PDF) ISBN 978-1-80355-770-0
ISSN 2631-5343

IntechOpen Book Series

Biomedical Engineering

Volume 13

Aims and Scope of the Series

Biomedical Engineering is one of the fastest-growing interdisciplinary branches of science and industry. The combination of electronics and computer science with biology and medicine has improved patient diagnosis, reduced rehabilitation time, and helped to facilitate a better quality of life. Nowadays, all medical imaging devices, medical instruments, or new laboratory techniques result from the cooperation of specialists in various fields. The series of Biomedical Engineering books covers such areas of knowledge as chemistry, physics, electronics, medicine, and biology. This series is intended for doctors, engineers, and scientists involved in biomedical engineering or those wanting to start working in this field.

Meet the Series Editor

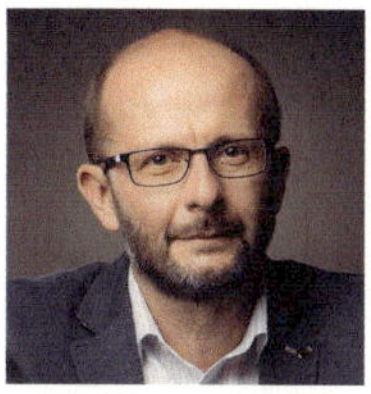

Robert Koprowski, MD (1997), Ph.D. (2003), Habilitation (2015), is an employee of the University of Silesia, Poland, Institute of Computer Science, Department of Biomedical Computer Systems. For 20 years, he has studied the analysis and processing of biomedical images, emphasizing the full automation of measurement for a large inter-individual variability of patients. Dr. Koprowski has authored more than a hundred research papers with dozens in impact factor (IF) journals and has authored or co-authored six books. Additionally, he is the author of several national and international patents in the field of biomedical devices and imaging. Since 2011, he has been a reviewer of grants and projects (including EU projects) in biomedical engineering.

Meet the Volume Editor

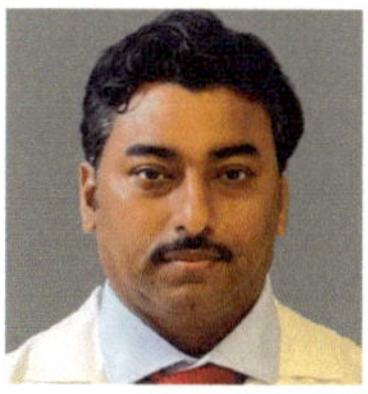

Manash K. Paul is a scientist and Principal Investigator at the University of California Los Angeles. He has contributed significantly to the fields of stem cell biology, regenerative medicine, and lung cancer. His research focuses on various signaling processes involved in maintaining stem cell homeostasis during the injury-repair process, deciphering the lung stem cell niche, pulmonary disease modeling, immuno-oncology, and drug discovery. He is currently investigating the role of extracellular vesicles in premalignant lung cell migration and detecting the metastatic phenotype of lung cancer via artificial intelligence-based analyses of exosomal Raman signatures. Dr. Paul also works on spatial multiplex immunofluorescence-based tissue mapping to understand the immune repertoire in lung cancer. Dr. Paul has published in more than sixty-five peer-reviewed international journals and is highly cited. He is the recipient of many awards, including the UCLA Vice Chancellor's award and the 2022 AAISCR-R Vijayalaxmi Award for Innovative Cancer Research. He is a senior member of the Institute of Electrical and Electronics Engineers (IEEE) and an editorial board member for several international journals.

Contents

Preface **XIII**

Section 1
Introduction **1**

Chapter 1 **3**
Introductory Chapter: Organoid Technology and Potential Applications
by Manash K. Paul

Section 2
Cerebral Organoid **9**

Chapter 2 **11**
Applications of Neural Organoids in Neurodevelopment and Regenerative Medicine
by Jing Gong, Jiahui Kang, Minghui Li, Xiao Liu, Jun Yang and Haiwei Xu

Chapter 3 **27**
The Brain Organoid Technology: Diversity of Protocols and Challenges
by Andrey Popatansov

Section 3
Retinal Organoid **51**

Chapter 4 **53**
Retinal Organoids over the Decade
by Jing Yuan and Zi-Bing Jin

Section 4
Organoid and Cancer **81**

Chapter 5 **83**
Evolution of Organoids in Oncology
by Allen Thayakumar Basanthakumar, Janitha Chandrasekhar Darlybai and Jyothsna Ganesh

Section 5
Organoid and Commercialization **103**

Chapter 6 **105**
Organoids and Commercialization
by Anubhab Mukherjee, Aprajita Sinha, Maheshree Maibam, Bharti Bisht and Manash K. Paul

Preface

Organoids are tiny in vitro 3D models that imitate the architecture and functioning of specific tissues and organs. These near-physiological models provide unique prospects for different fundamental and translational applications in human research. Organoid technology is a multidisciplinary technique that utilizes stem cells' ability to self-renew, differentiate into many lineages, and self-organize into organoids. Scientists have used organoid bioengineering techniques and explored the use of induced pluripotent stem cells (iPSCs), embryonic stem cells (ESCs), and tissue-resident adult stem cells (ASCs) in an attempt to create small tissue-replicating organoids. Several research teams have now manipulated stem cells in vitro to derive endodermal, mesodermal, and ectodermal organoids. Technological advances have made it possible to generate several tissue-specific organoids, including the kidney, brain, lung, colon, intestine, breast, retina, and liver. Considering the disparity between animal-based models and human disease pathology, a paradigm shift was needed to imitate human diseases correctly. The 3D human organoid platform offers an unparalleled chance to generate better models and a deeper understanding of human disease pathophysiology. Organoids give information on human disease-associated processes like disease-specific altered signaling, cell–cell interactions, therapeutic target identification, therapeutic screening, and discovery.

Advances in genome editing, hybrid culture techniques, single-cell transcriptomics, the establishment of biobanks, 3D printing, microfluidics, high-resolution imaging, nanotechnology, and other cutting-edge technologies are facilitating the development of physiologically accurate human disease models, hence impacting the discovery of new treatments. The combination of these approaches has the potential to push the limits of present scientific study, and future developments will undoubtedly lead to the development of new paradigms for treating human diseases. Tumor organoids are 3D cultures of cancer cells that may be successfully generated from individual patients. This facilitates the construction of a genetic mutation-specific tumoroid biobank with relevant patient samples that can be used for drug screening and development. Due to advances in biobanking, it is now feasible to use a person's stem cells or tumor cells for customized disease modeling and personalized therapy. Organoid-based disease modeling is a rapidly emerging field with enormous promise for revolutionary research possibilities, including preclinical research and theranostics. This collection of chapters aims to shed light on the expanding resources addressing the principles of organoids and disease modeling, including cancer. The primary areas covered in this book are organ-specific organoids, patient-derived organoids, tumoroids, and organoid commercialization. The chapters in this collection are intended for biologists, clinicians, and translational scientists.

Manash K. Paul
Department of Pulmonary and Critical Care Medicine,
University of California Los Angeles (UCLA),
Los Angeles, USA

Section 1

Introduction

Chapter 1

Introductory Chapter: Organoid Technology and Potential Applications

Manash K. Paul

1. Introduction

Owing to the fantastic potential of pluripotent stem cells (PSCs) to develop into all cell types in the body, regulating the differentiation of PSCs into particular tissue types is a substantial challenge. Early attempts to differentiate human PSCs (hPSCs) used two-dimensional (2D) monolayer cultures, resulting in cells that showed germ layer markers but lacked tissue architecture [1, 2]. Because of the potential to generate differentiated cells for therapeutic applications, human-induced pluripotent stem cells (iPSCs) are being researched more and more in stem cell research [3, 4]. Recent research has concentrated on developing organoids from human iPSCs and avoiding the ethical problems connected with embryonic stem cell (ESC) usage. Initial attempts at three-dimensional (3D) structure generation relied heavily on aggregation and spontaneous differentiation, resulting in disorganized tissue mixes [4, 5]. Recently, incredible progress has been made in the *in vitro* development of 3D organized tissues—dubbed organoids. Organoid technology is a multidisciplinary technique that uses stem cells' ability to self-renew, differentiate into many lineages, and self-organize into organoids. Scientists have explored human PSCs and adult stem cells (ASCs) to create tiny tissue mimics that resemble a wide variety of organs [6]. Several research groups have now manipulated PSCs and ASCs *in vitro* to generate endodermal, mesodermal, and ectodermal cell-derived organoids. Organoid culture has been used to promote the development of various tissues, including the kidney, brain, lung, colon, stomach, breast, liver, etc. (**Figure 1**).

Organoid technology has the potential to produce organ-specific tissue organoids and can provide an unprecedented opportunity for effective modeling of human-specific disease and to simulate the physiology and complexity of tissue-specific ailments. Given the existing difference between animal models and human disease pathology, a paradigm shift was needed to model human diseases appropriately. The 3D human organoid platform can aid in acquiring a better knowledge of the pathobiology of human diseases [7]. Organoids throw light on human disease-associated signaling interactions, cell-cell communications, therapeutic target identification, therapeutic discovery, and screening, thereby decoding the process of disease development in humans. Organoids closely replicates human physiology and simulates disorders affecting many organ systems is a more viable alternative to *in vivo* animal models when studying regenerative medicine [8]. It has now become feasible to use a person's own stem cells for personalized disease models and precision treatment as a result of improvements in biobanking [9, 10]. This collection of chapters attempts to bring together professionals from a variety of fields in order to shed light on the use of organoids in human disease management.

IntechOpen

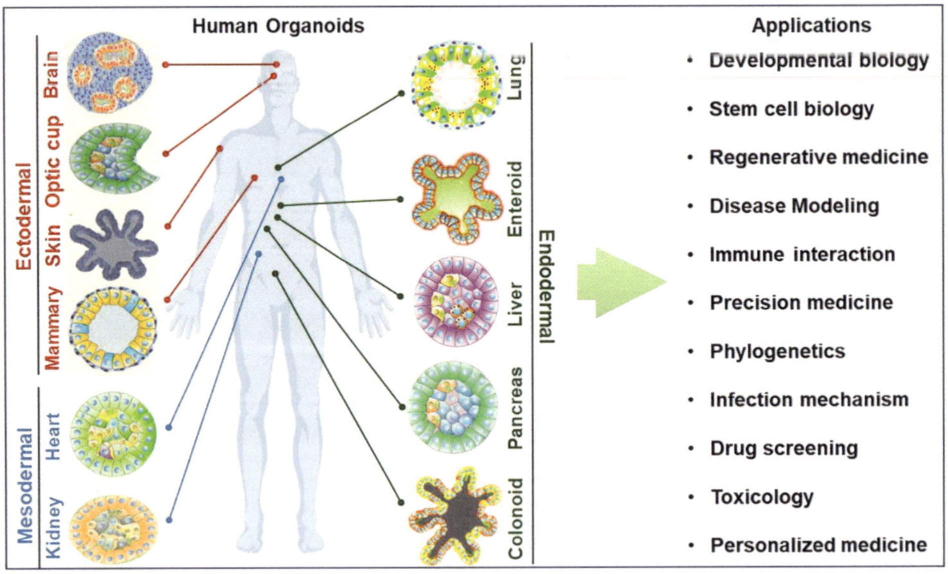

Figure 1.
Human organoids are vital in the progress of human biology research, preclinical investigations, and their translation into successful therapeutics.

Organoid-based disease modeling is a rapidly evolving field with significant potential for integrating novel techniques into future investigations [6]. Recent breakthroughs in organoid technology, such as creating a unique organoid platform, the engineering of organoid complexity, and the incorporation of pathological characteristics, have accelerated the development of tiny tissue or organs on a dish. Novel technologies, such as high-resolution 3D imaging, organ on a chip, 3D printing, gene manipulation, and single-cell sequencing, have accelerated the development of organoids, which can provide unprecedented insight into the behavior of stem cells, as well as serve as a platform for preclinical research and theranostics [11, 12]. Genome editing, hybrid culture techniques, biobank development, and single-cell sequencing are all examples of cutting-edge technologies that may help generate more physiologically realistic human disease models, thereby altering the identification of new therapies. A combination of these approaches has the potential to push the frontiers of present scientific study, and future advances will almost certainly result in the development of new paradigms for battling human diseases [7, 12]. This book presents a comprehensive overview of organoids and has three sections: Organ-specific organoid, Patient-derived organoid and tumoroid, and Organoid commercialization.

2. Organ-specific organoid

This section reviews how scientists are cultivating organ-specific tissue from stem cells, which has the potential to revolutionize the way diseases are investigated and treated. Retinal organoids (ROs) are unique to several exciting organoid types. ROs are 3D tissue constructs made from ESCs or iPSCs and accurately reproduce the spatiotemporal differentiation of the retina, making them useful *in vitro* models of retinal development and retinal disease [13]. ROs, available since 2011, allowed researchers to study retinal development (especially light-sensitive photoreceptors), pathology, and regeneration. The ROs' differentiation efficiency and development degree have improved dramatically during the last decade and offer many applications, including disease modeling. This section also reviews the role of ROs in evaluating disease pathogenesis, medication screening, and retinal regeneration treatment [14]. Although ROs have a promising future, their lack of structure and function, differentiation and culture constraints, and embryonic retina differences remain unsolved. Neural organoids, or cerebral organoids, are 3D *in vitro* culture systems produced from hPSCs that mimic the human brain's development. Specific distinctions between animal and human neurodevelopment have led to a dearth of information about human neurogenesis and understanding the pathological aspect. This section describes the applications of neural organoids in neurodevelopment and regenerative medicine. Advances in stem cell technology and the advent of the human-specific 3D neural organoid model are now widely used to study a specific aspect of the human brain and neurodevelopment. They can be vital in developing more effective therapeutics and regenerative medicine applications [15]. This section reviews current developments and future directions in the brain and retinal organoid developments and their applications.

3. Patient-derived organoid and tumoroid

The current paradigm for preclinical cancer drug development entails extensive and expensive optimization for lead discovery, often using *in vitro* human-cancer-cell-based models or *in vivo* animal-based tumor models that do not closely mirror actual solid tumors and, therefore, with little translational value [16]. Multicellular cancer "oids," including tumoroids, spheroids, and organoids, can address the existing loopholes in conventional 2D human cancer cell cultures and *in vivo* animal-based cancer models. Cancer "oids" display physiologically relevant cell-cell and cell-matrix interactions, gene expression and signaling pathway profiles, heterogeneity, and structural complexity, all of which are the characteristics of *in vivo* malignancies [17]. When cultivated appropriately, tumoroids develop easily and exhibit the *in vitro* model system's efficacy, repeatability, and resilience. Preclinical researchers are using tumoroids to present case studies on basic tumor biology, host-tumor interactions, and the application of high-throughput screening platforms for anticancer drug discovery and development [18]. This section discusses the evolution of organoids and research trends in cancer research.

This section also reviews patient-derived organoids (PDOs) as a revolutionary model system for cancer research. To circumvent the limitations of established cell lines, PDOs have recently been produced from varied tumor types [18, 19]. Researchers standardized 3D organoid culture methods to expand epithelial stem cells further and differentiate them into genetically and phenotypically stable "mini-organs in a dish," not only for humans but also for other species [17]. The *in vitro* response of PDOs mimics that of the result of related patients [20]. PDOs might be used to test immunomodulatory drugs in co-culture with different immune cell types. This book also addresses significant organoid-based bench-to-bedside applications and provides an overview of the therapeutic areas where organoids transform drug discovery and development.

4. Organoid commercialization

Organoids are 3D microtissue replicators that have been successfully employed for various applications, including disease modeling, drug screening, pathogenesis research, stem cell research, and tumor immunology. Organoids are as diverse as the tissues and organs of the human body and have immense economic potential [21, 22]. They have the potential to pave the path for personalized treatment and precision medicine (**Figure 1**). PDOs have been utilized in clinical trials to predict patient responses to therapy regimens and perhaps enhance cancer treatment results. Recent advances in stem cell research and genomic technology have resulted in ground-breaking breakthroughs in organoid bioengineering, large-scale production, biobanking, and commercialization [6]. This section of the book reviews the concept of organoid biobanking, the firms engaged, the commercialization process, and ethical issues. Additionally, this book discusses possible barriers to clinical translation of organoids and suggests future research avenues for therapeutic translation and cancer treatment. This collection of chapters is intended for a wide readership and will serve as an indispensable resource for fundamental biologists, translational scientists, and clinicians.

Author details

Manash K. Paul
Department of Pulmonary and Critical Care Medicine, David Geffen School of Medicine, University of California Los Angeles (UCLA), Los Angeles, California, USA

*Address all correspondence to: manashp@ucla.edu; paul_cancerbiotech@yahoo.co.in

References

[1] Kim J, Koo B-K, Knoblich JA. Human organoids: Model systems for human biology and medicine. Nature Reviews Molecular Cell Biology. 2020;**21**(10):571-584

[2] Mahapatra C, Lee R, Paul MK. Emerging role and promise of nanomaterials in organoid research. Drug Discovery Today. 2021;**27**(3):890-899

[3] Turhan AG, Hwang JW, Chaker D, Tasteyre A, Latsis T, Griscelli F, et al. iPSC-derived organoids as therapeutic models in regenerative medicine and oncology. Frontiers in Medicine. 2021;**8**:728543

[4] Orqueda AJ, Giménez CA, Pereyra-Bonnet F. iPSCs: A Minireview from bench to bed, including organoids and the CRISPR System. Stem Cells International. 2016;**2016**:1-9

[5] Takebe T, Wells JM, Helmrath MA, Zorn AM. Organoid center strategies for accelerating clinical translation. Cell Stem Cell. 2018;**22**(6):806-809

[6] Shen H. Core concept: Organoids have opened avenues into investigating numerous diseases. But how well do they mimic the real thing? Proceedings of the National Academy of Sciences. 2018;**115**(14):3507-3509

[7] Lancaster MA, Knoblich JA. Organogenesis in a dish: Modeling development and disease using organoid technologies. Science. 2014;**345**(6194):1247125

[8] Lee S-J, Lee H-A. Trends in the development of human stem cell-based non-animal drug testing models. The Korean Journal of Physiology & Pharmacology. 2020;**24**(6):441-452

[9] Yan HHN, Siu HC, Law S, Ho SL, Yue SSK, Tsui WY, et al. A comprehensive human gastric cancer organoid biobank captures tumor subtype heterogeneity and enables therapeutic screening. Cell Stem Cell. 2018;**23**(6):882-97.e11

[10] Wilkinson DC, Alva-Ornelas JA, Sucre JMS, Vijayaraj P, Durra A, Richardson W, et al. Development of a three-dimensional bioengineering technology to generate lung tissue for personalized disease modeling. Stem Cells Translational Medicine. 2017;**6**(2):622-633

[11] Wang Z, He X, Qiao H, Chen P. Global trends of organoid and organ-on-a-chip in the past decade: A bibliometric and comparative study. Tissue Engineering Part A. 2020;**26**(11-12):656-671

[12] Garreta E, Kamm RD, de Sousa C, Lopes SM, Lancaster MA, Weiss R, et al. Rethinking organoid technology through bioengineering. Nature Materials. 2020;**20**(2):145-155

[13] Fligor CM, Langer KB, Sridhar A, Ren Y, Shields PK, Edler MC, et al. Three-dimensional retinal organoids facilitate the investigation of retinal ganglion cell development, organization and neurite outgrowth from human pluripotent stem cells. Scientific Reports. 2018;**8**(1):14520

[14] Fathi M, Ross CT, Hosseinzadeh Z. Functional 3-dimensional retinal organoids: Technological progress and existing challenges. Frontiers in Neuroscience. 2021;**15**:668857

[15] Chhibber T, Bagchi S, Lahooti B, Verma A, Al-Ahmad A, Paul MK, et al. CNS organoids: An innovative tool for neurological disease modeling and drug

neurotoxicity screening. Drug Discovery Today. 2020;**25**(2):456-465

[16] Li YF, Gao Y, Liang BW, Cao XQ, Sun ZJ, Yu JH, et al. Patient-derived organoids of non-small cells lung cancer and their application for drug screening. Neoplasma. 2020;**67**(02):430-437

[17] Lee SH, Hu W, Matulay JT, Silva MV, Owczarek TB, Kim K, et al. Tumor evolution and drug response in patient-derived organoid models of bladder cancer. Cell. 2018;**173**(2):515-28.e17

[18] Jacob F, Salinas RD, Zhang DY, Nguyen PTT, Schnoll JG, Wong SZH, et al. A patient-derived glioblastoma organoid model and biobank recapitulates inter- and intra-tumoral heterogeneity. Cell. 2020;**180**(1):188-204.e22

[19] Fiorini E, Veghini L, Corbo V. Modeling cell communication in cancer with organoids: Making the complex simple. Frontiers in Cell and Developmental Biology. 2020;**8**:166

[20] Zhou Z, Cong L, Cong X. Patient-derived organoids in precision medicine: drug screening, organoid-on-a-chip and living organoid biobank. Frontiers in Oncology. 2021;**11**:762184

[21] Sachs N, de Ligt J, Kopper O, Gogola E, Bounova G, Weeber F, et al. A living biobank of breast cancer organoids captures disease heterogeneity. Cell. 2018;**172**(1-2):373-86.e10

[22] Choudhury D, Ashok A, Naing MW. Commercialization of organoids. Trends in Molecular Medicine. 2020;**26**(3):245-249

Section 2

Cerebral Organoid

Chapter 2

Applications of Neural Organoids in Neurodevelopment and Regenerative Medicine

Jing Gong, Jiahui Kang, Minghui Li, Xiao Liu, Jun Yang and Haiwei Xu

Abstract

Recent advances in stem cell technologies have enabled the application of three-dimensional neural organoids for exploring the mechanisms of neurodevelopment and regenerative medicine. Over the past decade, series of studies have been carried out to investigate the cellular and molecular events of human neurogenesis using animal models, while the species differences between animal models and human being prevent a full understanding of human neurogenesis. Human neural organoids provide a new model system for gaining a more complete understanding of human neural development and their applications in regenerative medicine. In this chapter, the recent advances of the neural organoids of the brain and retina as well as their applications in neurodevelopment and regenerative medicine are reviewed.

Keywords: neural organoids, neurogenesis, brain, retina, neurodevelopment, regenerative medicine

1. Introduction

Researchers have been attracted by the mystery of human neural development for hundreds of years. Numerous cellular and animal models have been explored to improve our understanding of neurogenesis in humans for hundreds of years. Although animal models have greatly improved our understanding of neural development, neurological disorders, cortical architecture, and functional regionalization, there are significant differences between the human and rodent brains. For example, the organization and behavior of neural progenitors during embryonic development determine the expansion and folding of the human neocortex to a large degree. Therefore, studying the development of the human brain requires models with human brain characteristics. Organoids are simply, self-organized three-dimensional (3D) tissue cultures that are derived from human pluripotent stem cells (hPSCs), including embryonic stem cells (ESCs) and induced pluripotent stem cells (iPSCs), which has gained great interest in simulating tissue development and disease. This technology opens a window to observe some of the most elusive aspects of human biology. Compared with animal models or two-dimensional (2D) cell culture systems,

3D-cultured organoids can overcome the differences between species and closely represent the realistic human-specific development features, which can be utilized to mimic the architecture and functionality of the human tissues, having great advantages in explaining the unique human developmental processes [1, 2]. In the field of neurodevelopment and regenerative medicine, neural organoids replicate human specific features of neurodevelopment, contributing to modeling neurogenesis and neurological diseases [3, 4]. Central nervous system (CNS) injury or damage initiates spatial and temporal neurodegeneration, resulting in irreversible neuronal loss and functional deficits. The vertebrate retina is an extension of the CNS that is composed of seven main types of neurons and glial cells. In recent years, emerging organoid-based research studies of brain and retina have made progress in understanding neural organogenesis, which facilitates successful application of 3D organoid systems in disease modeling and regenerative medicine. In this chapter, we summarize the application of neural organoids of the brain and retina in neurodevelopment and regenerative medicine.

2. Organoids in neural development

CNS is generally regarded as the most complex system in human body. Limited by accessibility of living neural tissues and ethical challenges, human-specific features of neurodevelopment and neurological diseases remain largely unknown to us. Recent advances in stem cell technologies and 3D culture neural organoids have opened a new avenue in exploring the mechanisms of neurodevelopment. Early versions of the neural organoids range from complex neural epithelial structures to disorganized brain regions with large cellular diversity [5]. By supplementing exogenous factors and assembly of organoids during embryonic brain development, efforts have been made to gain the well-developed multilayer neural organoids and higher-order functions in terms of controlling patterning, morphogenesis, and function [6, 7].

2.1 Neural organoids in brain development

Through the embryonic brain development, neural progenitors progressively follow precise orchestration and coordination to acquire their spatial identities, a process characterized by successive changes in cellular composition and cyto-architecture (**Figure 1a**). Dysregulation of this process may affect neurogenesis, synaptogenesis, and myelination and induce neurological or psychiatric disorders. To better investigate the early formation and function of the human brain *in vitro*, two different methodologies have been applied to generate human brain organoids: unguided and guided methods. The unguided methods rely largely on the capacity of spontaneous morphogenesis and intrinsic differentiation of the 3D aggregates while the guided organoid methods highly require supplementation of exogenous factors to induce hPSCs to differentiate toward specific brain regions [5]. Over the past decade, guided methods were induced by a set of growth factors and small molecules to induce the production of brain organs containing broad and specific identity, including forebrain, large cortical organoids, cerebellum, midbrain, and hippocampus. For instance, glycogen synthase kinase-3 (GSK-3) inhibitor, SMAD inhibitors, and WNT3A were for forebrain organoids induction [6]; SMAD inhibitors, Wnt activator, sonic hedgehog (SHH), and FGF8 were used for midbrain organoids induction [8]; FGF19 and SDF1 for cerebellum organoids induction [9]; WNT-3A and SHH were

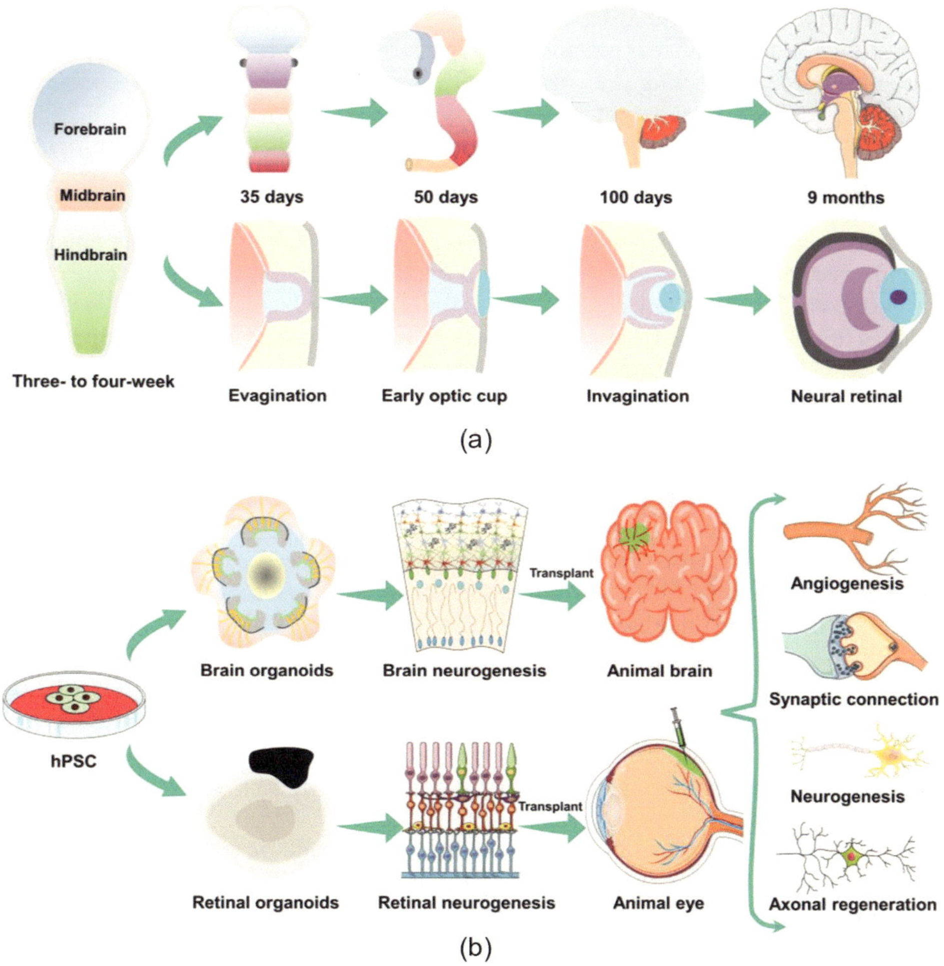

Figure 1.
Schematic depiction of brain and eye development in vivo and in vitro. a. The timeline of brain development in human body and the features of human retinal development. b. Generation of hPSC-derived human brain organoids and retinal organoids in vitro, and the application of the generated organoids in regenerative medicine.

used for hypothalamic organoids induction [10]. These generated brain organoids show robust neuronal and glial subtypes resembling the organization, transcriptional frameworks, and developmental timing of a primitive human fetal brain.

The 3D cultured brain organoids have been proven useful for many applications in basic research, for example, the development of the human brain cortex. It firstly begins with the expansion of the neuroepithelium, and then folds into six different layers. The main principles of the cortical layer formation are similar between mammals, such as primates and humans; however, the morphological differences are unneglectable. It is well known that neuronal number in primates massively increases in cortical surface, which eventually leads to the gyrification of the cortex (the generation of gyri and sulci) [11]. However, the mechanisms controlling the generation of gyrification are still not clear during the formation of cortical areas. The application of cortical organoids has helped us better understand the rapid expansion of human neocortex and the formation of cerebral cortical sulcus and gyrus. Karzbrun et al. revealed two opposing mechanical forces with the usage of the brain organoids-on-a-chip: the middle cytoskeletal contraction and peripheral cell-cycle-dependent nuclear expansion, physically leading to differential growth and folding into brain wrinkling [12], and the extracellular matrix (ECM) components are implicated in neocortical expansion [13].

For another example, brain organoids are used to investigate the development of cellular interactions in the human brain. The human CNS originated from several distinct vesicles and then after a range of progenitors migrate and integrate, it moves into areas to generate multiple intertwined regions, ultimately resulting in emerging complex networks, neurons branching, and projecting. To model the intricate cellular interactions in human brain, fusing regionalized organoids into assembloids recapitulates more elaborate biological processes of brain development. This approach has been applied to study forebrain axis establishment, interneuron migration, oligodendrogenesis, and neuronal projections like the fused dorsal-ventral cerebral organoids to model interneuron migration in [7, 14, 15].

2.2 Neural organoids in retinal development

The eye originates from the ventral diencephalon, where a group of eye field transcription factors (EFTFs) are highly expressed such as PAX6, RAX, SIX3, and OTX2, and becomes specified as the eye field [16]. The eye field region is firstly split into optic vesicles in pairs and subsequently forms the optic cup by experiencing the valgus and invagination of the optic vesicle. The outer layer of the optic cup develops into retinal pigment epithelium(RPE) while the inner layer develops into neural retina. The neural retina with multilayered structure undergoes different phases of development, with different types of cells differentiating and maturing over the time (**Figure 1a**).

However, the understandings of the function and development of the human retinal are limited by scarce human fetal retina sample and species differences between animals and human. Since 2011, Sasai et al. released a landmark study to generate a self-organized 3D optic cup with layered neuroepithelia from mouse pluripotent stem cells (mPSCs), which opened a window for generating retinal models [17]. Many research groups have subsequently optimized the protocol to generate human retinal organoids derived from hPSCs. During retinal organoid generation, stem cell patterns the eye field-like regions expressing a complete component of the EFTFs to mimic the optic vesicle in early development [18]. What is encouraging, these tiny retinal organoids even contain almost all relevant retinal cell types: retinal ganglion cells (RGCs), amacrine cells, horizontal cells, bipolar cells, Müller cells, and photoreceptors.

2.2.1 Retinal organoids in RGC development

RGCs, the early-born neurons, transmit visual information between the eye and the brain, playing a critical role in retinal neuronal outputs. The loss of RGCs trends to result in a group of degenerative diseases such as glaucoma and optic nerve hypoplasia. Due to the specific time point of the RGC development, it is a challenge to obtain human fetus samples. In addition, the long-distance projection of neurites is the mostly important characteristic for RGC development as the extension of axons is regulated by extrinsic factors, including the ECM, growth factors, and glial cells. Recent several approaches have improved the capacity to differentiate hPSC-derived retinal organoids into RGCs that possess appropriate morphological and functional properties [19]. For example, Fligor et al. found that substrate composition including laminin and Matrigel shows the most conducive for RGC neurite outgrowth; similarly, the growth factors with Netrin-1 and BDNF have the ability to guide and direct RGC axons outgrowth [20]. Besides, single-cell RNA sequencing (RNA-seq) results proved that the ganglion cells of retinal organoids at day 60 give the similar clusters to the human fetal retina on day 59 [21]. Collectively, the established retinal organoids serve as effective models for investigations of RGC development and disease modeling and as a valuable tool for cell replacement.

2.2.2 Retinal organoids in photoreceptors development

Rod and cone photoreceptors are specialized neurons with functioning in the initial step of vision, which convert light stimuli into neurological responses. Rods are highly sensitive to light and operate under dim lighting conditions while the cones control color vision and high visual acuity. It is reported that the progressive loss of photoreceptors leads to blindness-associated inherited retinal diseases(IRDs), such as well-known retinitis pigmentosa (RP), congenital stationary night blindness(CSNB), and Leber congenital amaurosis (LCA). Therefore, it is particularly important to understand retinal progenitor fate choices toward rod photoreceptors and cone subtypes during retinogenesis. As such, the phototransduction mechanism requires a complicated cascade of gene regulatory networks. Aiming to induce hPCS-derived retinal organoids with mature photoreceptors, efforts of genetic manipulation and transcriptomic analysis have become the focal point for researchers [22]. Most recently, NRL (neural retina leucine zipper)$^{-/-}$ human-based 3D organoids were used to uncover the regulative role of MEF2C in cones' development [22]. RNAseq analysis of hPCS-derived retinal organoids has identified certain molecular signatures related with human photoreceptors development [23]. In brief, these observations and datasets have enabled to reconstruct developmental trajectories and recapitulate dynamics *in vivo* photoreceptors development.

3. Neural organoids in regenerative medicine

Neural organoids, which recapitulate the process of native neurogenesis in the development of CNS, have been applied in a large variety of areas including simulating brain development and retinogenesis. Moreover, emerging organoid-based cell transplantation has made considerable progress in reconstruction of lost neural circuits, damaged neural cortex and visual function, which facilitates the application of 3D organoid systems in disease modeling and regenerative medicine. Representative examples are involved in two aspects: (a) isolating neural progenitor cells (NPCs) from neural organoids; (b) transplanting neural organoids in immunodeficient animals. The stem cells in the organoids derived from hPSCs present a higher survival rate and closer connection with the surrounding tissues in the host. Distinct from conventional stem cell therapy usually focusing on specific populations of stem cells or NPCs, neural organoids offer an entire set of cell types of the human organs.

3.1 Brain organoid system in regenerative medicine

Brain disorders, such as Alzheimer's disease (AD), Parkinson's disease (PD), traumatic brain injury (TBI), and stroke, along with several other chronic neurodegenerative disorders, are debilitating diseases that have few treatment options. Stem cell therapy is likely to provide beneficial effects for the indications of these diseases. The current understanding of brain diseases is mainly based on traditional 2D monocultural cells, animal models, and postmortem examination. Because of the inherent species differences between animals and humans and the individual differences among genetic and environmental backgrounds, it remains a challenge to investigate brain development and associated disorders. To establish better models of human brain development, stem-cell-based 3D brain organoids systematically decipher the developmental rules, presenting the 3D architectures and physiology of the brain. These generated brain organoids show robust neuronal subtypes and glial subtypes and functionality to mimic *in vivo* neural connectivity [24, 25]. In comparison with 2D monocultural stem cell cultures, physiologic conditions closer to the human organism are provided by organoids to support cell-cell and cell-matrix interactions. Therefore, as an ideal cell source, brain organoids have great potential for the reconstruction of lost neural circuits. Brain organoids transplantation strategy is expected to become an effective treatment for neurological defects after brain injury (**Figure 1b**).

Recently, in two studies, scientists transplanted hPSC-derived cerebral organoids into mouse cerebral cortex and successfully generated vascularized organoids, which promoted the progressive neuronal differentiation and maturation and increased cell survival [26, 27]. They observed the widespread axonal extension and precise synaptic connectivity outside the graft area; however, the region-specific long projections and synaptogenesis mapping were not reported in the two studies. Previously, reported approaches produced brain organoids with large lumens and tubes, which results in insufficient oxygen and nutrients support in increasing metabolic needs, making them difficult to apply in transplantation therapy [10, 28]. Recently, an optimized culture protocol was developed to efficiently generate small human cerebral organoids, which presents the benefit of alleviating the risk of cell overgrowth and safety concerns after injecting into the mouse medial prefrontal cortex [29]. The transplanted cerebral organoids extended projections to basal brain regions and generated human glutamatergic neurons with mature electrophysiology [29]. Moreover, mice transplanted with cerebral organoids show potentiated auditory startle fear response, indicating that the organoids can be functionally integrated into preexisting host mouse neural circuits via building up bidirectional synaptic connections, which provides crucial therapeutic strategy for neurological diseases [29].

However, owing to the cellular composition of brain, organoids dramatically changes along the time course of the development, it is necessary to demonstrate which stage of the organoids is best suitable for transplantation. To address this limitation, Kitahara et al. transplanted hESC-derived cerebral organoids at 6w or 10w into mouse cerebral cortex and found that 6w-organoids extend more axons along corticospinal tracts but caused graft overgrowth with higher populations of proliferative cells while axonal extensions from 10w-organoids were smaller in number but enhanced after brain injury 1 week [30]. A similar study reported that 55d and 85d-cerebral organoids were transplanted into damaged motor cortex, indicating that 55d-cerebral organoids can be used as a better transplantation donor for traumatic brain injury (TBI) [31]. Cells from the transplanted cerebral organoids have the capability to support region-specific reconstruction of damaged brain cortex, upregulate hippocampal neural connection protein and neurotrophic factor, and improve of damaged motor cortex. It is also reported that cerebral organoids were transplanted at 55 days to explore the feasibility of organoid transplantation in stroke [32]. Cerebral organoids were transplanted at 6 h or 24 h after middle cerebral artery occlusion (MCAO) surgery, resulting in reducing brain infarct volume and improving neurological motor function. Furthermore, they also observed that the transplanted cerebral organoids were also related with increased neurogenesis, synaptic reconstruction, axonal regeneration and angiogenesis, decreased neural apoptosis, and rescued more survival neurons after stroke [32]. Although a few works with respect to transplanting brain organoid system were reported, it still has promising technologies in the future treatment of central nervous system diseases. Hence, the effects of the developmental organoid stage and host brain environment should be accurately evaluated when developing an organoid-replacement therapy for brain injury.

3.2 Retinal organoid in regenerative medicine

Retinal degenerative diseases, such as glaucoma, RP, and Age-Related Macular Degeneration (AMD), usually lead to irreversible blindness. So does the importance of finding a viable treatment. Regardless of the underlying etiology of retinal degeneration, the common endpoint is the loss of photoreceptors and underlying RPE. Cell replacement strategy provides a good solution for the treatment of retinal degeneration. Although plenty of studies have been made to understand the cellular and molecular mechanisms of retinal disorders, our knowledge is still in its infancy, and the immortalized retinal cell lines have not recapitulated the developmental stages of the human native retina. The new methodological advances in inducing hPSCs into human retina tissues have opened new possibilities for basic research on investigating the therapies or treatments in regenerative medicine [18, 33]. The generated retinal organoids closely resemble many aspects of the real human retina, including retina-specific ribbon synapse [34] and physiological-relevant response to light stimuli [35], which empower researchers to explore the pathogenesis of retinal diseases and pursue cell/tissue transplantation for developing novel treatment options. Because retinal organoids contain all the cell types of human retina, it plays a primary role in the field of transplantation therapy. In this section, we focus on single-cell suspensions isolated from retinal organoids and application of retinal organoids sheets transplantation used for cell therapies in regenerative medicine (**Figure 1b**).

3.2.1 Retinal organoids as a cell source for therapeutic transplantation

During the previous decade, the aborted human fetal tissues and the hPSC-derived retinal progenitors were two cell sources for transplantation. Representative retinal cell replacement clinical trials are transplantation of hPSC-derived RPE for the treatment of retinal diseases, including AMD and Stargardt disease [36–38]. It has been proved that the mature mammalian retina lacks the ability to accept and incorporate stem cells or to promote photoreceptor differentiation. In 2006, stem-cell-derived precursor photoreceptors were first integrated into the outer retinal layer of degenerating retina and had success in improving vision [39, 40]. However, the strong ethical restrictions and limited cell sources remain a challenge in current transplantation therapies. The retinal organoids that contain abundant retinal progenitor cells (RPCs) can act as an ideal cell source transplantation in retinal degenerative diseases. Zou et al. transplanted effectively purifying RPCs with the surface markers (C-Kit+/SSEA4−) into the retinal degeneration models of rats and mice, showing benefits to the improvement of vision and preservation of the retinal structure [41]. The RGCs are the earliest differentiated cells closely associated with glaucoma. But the population of RGCs in retinal organoids is not substantial as they gradually degenerate following long-term culture time. Thus, prolonging the survival time of RGCs may provide the possibility for RGC replacement therapy. Several approaches have been taken to improve the short life of implanted RGCs and the length of axons, such as adding extrinsic growth factors [20], combining 2D and 3D protocols [42], and co-culturing with Müller glia [43]. In another animal study, by transplanting purified rod photoreceptors isolated from retinal organoids in defective S- and M- cone opsins, $Nrl^{-/-}$ mouse retinas can restore rod-mediated visual function and be incorporated into the host retina with forming synaptic-like structures in close apposition to mouse interneurons [44]. Interestingly, recent studies contradicted the common view that transplanted photoreceptors integrate into the photoreceptor layer of recipients. They demonstrated that the material transfer between donor rod photoreceptors and host photoreceptors leads to the acquisition of proteins originally expressed only by donor cells [45, 46]. Thus, the mechanism of the photoreceptor transplantation demands reinterpretation.

3.2.2 Retinal organoid sheet transplantation for improving visual function

A retinal sheet derived from cultured retinal organoids or fetal retina is another approach to preserving the neural circuitries and improving visual function. Cell suspension strategies consist of transplanting purified photoreceptor precursor cells, whereas retinal sheet transplantations engraft retinal organoids containing both photoreceptor cells and inner retinal neurons. The inner neurons located in the transplanted retinal sheet, which serves as a scaffold and nurturing microenvironment, are conductive to outer layer retinal cells in differentiation and maturation, preserving normal lamination structures. It is reported that the retinal sheet graft can produce less immune activation that enhances life span and the survival rate of transplanted cells, providing suitability approach for therapies of late-stage retinal diseases.

Furthermore, several studies have demonstrated that the transplantation of hPSC-derived RPE cells in AMD patients shows promising outcomes in clinical trials, such as improvement in retinal integrity, maintainability in visual acuity, and increase in vision-related quality of life [47]. Currently, the transplantation of early-stage retinal organoid sheets is verified to establish connections more effectively with host retinal degeneration, and these connections show higher survival rate over time. A series of studies have been performed to investigate whether the transplantation of retinal organoid sheets can differentiate, integrate, and improve visual function in animal models with severe retinal degeneration [48–50]. In 2016, Shirai et al. dissected "retinas" from organoids to get transparent and continuous neural retina sheets and transplanted them into two primate models with retinal degeneration. In both monkey and rat, grafted hESC-retina differentiated into a range of retinal cell types, such as photoreceptors. The photoreceptors were proved to have migrated to the outer nuclear layer and the host-graft synaptic connections were established in those animal models [51]. Similar results were achieved in another study of transplanting the sheets dissected from hESC-derived retinal organoids into retinal degenerate rats [48]. In addition, to enhance functional integration of transplanted retinal sheet, a method in which a genetic modification was used to reduce ON-bipolar cells resulted in efficiently restoring RGC light responsiveness in degenerated retina [52]. However, in those studies, the absence of a well-defined RPE monolayer presents a main limiting factor for retinal sheet transplantation. To overcome this limitation, hESC-derived retinal organoids and RPE monolayer were combined using different bio-adhesives to transplant into immunodeficient Royal College of Surgeons (RCS) rats. The co-grafts were observed to reconstruct the severely damaged retina structure and improve visual function [53]. Those studies demonstrate the clinical feasibility of hPSC-derived retinal organoids sheet transplantation and provide practical tools to optimize transplantation strategies for future clinical applications.

In retinal tissue engineering, biomaterials are utilized to optimize the models of the human retina. A growing number of biomaterials, especially synthetic polymer scaffolds, such as biodegradable polycaprolactone (PCL) and polylactic-coglycolic acid (PLGA), have been widely used. The remarkable properties of defined synthetic polymer substrate are thin and biodegradable, which can be placed into the retinal subretinal space with minimal physical distortion [54]. In terms of the report, transplanting mouse RPCs cultured on biodegradable thin-film PCL scaffolds with varying surface topographies into the retinal subretinal space help newly integrated mRPCs exhibit potential to guide stem cell differentiation toward photoreceptor fate and to help cells localized to the outer nuclear layer [55]. Another study implanted the human retinal organoids, which are seeded on PLGA sheets into both normal and Chronic Ocular Hypertension (OHT) rhesus monkey retinas. They found that despite the need of immunosuppression for dexamethasone after transplantation, survival and differentiation into retinal tissue were successfully improved [56]. Subsequently, the same group proved again that with the support of PLGA sheets, retinal organoids showed active proliferation, migration and projection of axons into the host optic nerve after transplanting into OHT rhesus monkey eyes [57].

4. Comments and future challenges

Development of neural organoid techniques has yielded rapid progress in clarifying the mechanisms of human neural development. Organoids display many characteristics of the organs from which they were made, including cellular anatomy and interaction, genetics, and specific tissue functions, advancing our understanding the neuro of biology, developmental science, and regeneration. Some of the limitations and challenges of neural organoids have been addressed, but emerging technologies are still required to be applied in further study. With respect to brain organoids, many points are needed to be improved, such as the maturation of neuronal and glial cells, reliable anatomical organization, long-range axonal projection and synaptic connections, and the precise construction of neuronal circuits. Providing a physiologically relevant microenvironment and the more complex whole-brain organoids to reproduce the developmental events of the human nervous systems may be needed in the future. Retinal organoids serve as an ideal choice for therapeutic transplantation, which still face many challenges as following: low yield, high heterogeneity, degenerative inner cell layers, and cancerogenesis. The next-generation retinal organoids would be anticipated to have an integrated vascular network, mature microglia system, and pigment layer wrapping around as well as the integration of bioengineering technologies. To achieve the goal, several engineering approaches may be useful: (1) engineered biomaterials to investigate cell-cell and cell-matrix interactions; (2) genetic engineering technology to study various aspects of organoids development and performance; (3) organoid-on-a-chip device to create an optimal microenvironment with the purpose of generating organoids with higher physiological relevance. Furthermore, the next generation of organoids probably needs to integrate more bioengineering technologies, aiming to overcome each approach's limitation and provide a superior, synergistic approach for constructing more complex organoids in regenerative and precision medicine.

Declaration of competing interest

The authors declare no conflicts of interest.

Acknowledgements

This study was supported by the funding from the National Key Research and Development Program of China (Grant No. 2018YFA0107302); the National Natural Science Foundation of China (Grant No. 31930068); and the Military Key Program (Grant No. 20QNPY025).

Author details

Jing Gong[1,2,3], Jiahui Kang[1,2], Minghui Li[1,2], Xiao Liu[1,2], Jun Yang[3] and Haiwei Xu[1,2*]

1 Southwest Hospital/Southwest Eye Hospital, Third Military Medical University (Army Medical University), Chongqing, China

2 Key Lab of Visual Damage and Regeneration and Restoration of Chongqing, Chongqing, China

3 Key Laboratory of Biorheological Science and Technology, Ministry of Education, College of Bioengineering, Chongqing University, Chongqing, China

*Address all correspondence to: haiweixu2001@163.com

References

[1] Shi YC, Wu Q, Wang XQ. Modeling brain development and diseases with human cerebral organoids. Current Opinion in Neurobiology. 2021;**66**:103-115. DOI: 10.1016/j.conb.2020.09.006

[2] O'Hara-Wright M, Gonzalez-Cordero A. Retinal organoids: A window into human retinal development. Development. 2020;**147**:dev189746. DOI: 10.1242/dev.189746

[3] Chhibber T, Bagchi S, Lahooti B, Verma A, Al-Ahmad A, Paul MK, et al. CNS organoids: An innovative tool for neurological disease modeling and drug neurotoxicity screening. Drug Discovery Today. 2020;**25**:456-465. DOI: 10.1016/j.drudis.2019.11.010

[4] Lu X, Yang J, Xiang Y. Modeling human neurodevelopmental diseases with brain organoids. Cell Regeneration. 2022;**11**:1. DOI: 10.1186/s13619-021-00103-6

[5] Lancaster MA, Renner M, Martin CA, Wenzel D, Bicknell LS, Hurles ME, et al. Cerebral organoids model human brain development and microcephaly. Nature. 2013;**501**:373-379. DOI: 10.1038/nature12517

[6] Qian XY, Nguyen HN, Song MM, Hadiono C, Ogden SC, Hammack C, et al. Brain-region-specific organoids using mini-bioreactors for modeling ZIKV exposure. Cell. 2016;**165**:1238-1254. DOI: 10.1016/j.cell.2016.04.032

[7] Bagley JA, Reumann D, Bian S, Levi-Strauss J, Knoblich JA. Fused cerebral organoids model interactions between brain regions. Nature Methods. 2017;**14**:743-751. DOI: 10.1038/nmeth.4304

[8] Jo J, Xiao YX, Sun AX, Cukuroglu E, Tran HD, Goke J, et al. Midbrain-like organoids from human pluripotent stem cells contain functional dopaminergic and neuromelanin-producing neurons. Cell Stem Cell. 2016;**19**:248-2457. DOI: 10.1016/j.stem.2016.07.005

[9] Muguruma K, Nishiyama A, Kawakami H, Hashimoto K, Sasai Y. Self-organization of polarized cerebellar tissue in 3D culture of human pluripotent stem cells. Cell Reports. 2015;**10**:537-550. DOI: 10.1016/j.celrep.2014.12.051

[10] Qian XY, Jacob F, Song MM, Nguyen HN, Song HJ, Ming GL. Generation of human brain region-specific organoids using a miniaturized spinning bioreactor. Nature Protocols. 2018;**13**:565-580. DOI: 10.1038/nprot.2017.152

[11] Kyrousi C, Cappello S. Using brain organoids to study human neurodevelopment, evolution and disease. WIREs Developmental Biology. 2020;**9**:e347. DOI: 10.1002/wdev.347

[12] Karzbrun E, Kshirsagar A, Cohen SR, Hanna JH, Reiner O. Human brain organoids on a chip reveal the physics of folding. Nature Physics. 2018;**14**:515-522. DOI: 10.1038/s41567-018-0046-7

[13] Long KR, Newland B, Florio M, Kalebic N, Langen B, Kolterer A, et al. Extracellular matrix components HAPLN1, lumican, and collagen I cause hyaluronic acid-dependent folding of the developing human Neocortex. Neuron. 2018;**99**:702-719. DOI: 10.1016/j.neuron.2018.07.013

[14] Birey F, Andersen J, Makinson CD, Islam S, Wei W, Huber N, et al. Assembly of functionally integrated human forebrain spheroids. Nature. 2017;**545**:54-59. DOI: 10.1038/nature22330

[15] Xiang YF, Tanaka Y, Patterson B, Kang YJ, Govindaiah G, Roselaar N, et al. Fusion of regionally specified hPSC-derived organoids models human brain development and interneuron migration. Cell Stem Cell. 2017;**21**:383-398. DOI: 10.1016/j.stem.2017.07.007

[16] Vielle A, Park YK, Secora C, Vergara MN. Organoids for the study of retinal development and developmental Aabnormalities. Frontiers in Cellular Neuroscience. 2021;**15**:667880. DOI: 10.3389/fncel.2021.667880

[17] Eiraku M, Takata N, Ishibashi H, Kawada M, Sakakura E, et al. Self-organizing optic-cup morphogenesis in three-dimensional culture. Nature. 2011;**472**:51-56. DOI: 10.1038/nature09941

[18] Zhong XF, Gutierrez C, Xue T, Hampton C, Vergara MN, Cao LH, et al. Generation of three-dimensional retinal tissue with functional photoreceptors from human iPSCs. Nature Communications. 2014;**5**:4047. DOI: 10.1038/ncomms5047

[19] Aparicio JG, Hopp H, Choi A, Comar JM, Liao VC, Harutyunyan N, et al. Temporal expression of CD184(CXCR4) and CD171(L1CAM) identifies distinct early developmental stages of human retinal ganglion cells in embryonic stem cell derived retina. Experimental Eye Research. 2017;**154**:177-189. DOI: 10.1016/j.exer.2016.11.013

[20] Fligor CM, Langer KB, Sridhar A, Ren Y, Shields PK, Edler MC, et al. Three-dimensional retinal organoids facilitate the investigation of retinal ganglion cell development, organization and neurite outgrowth from human pluripotent stem cells. Scientific Reports. 2018;**8**:14520. DOI: 10.1038/s41598-018-32871-8

[21] Sridhar A, Hoshino A, Finkbeiner CR, Chitsazan A, Dai L, Haugan AK, et al. Single-cell transcriptomic comparison of human fetal retina, hPSC-derived retinal organoids, and long-term retinal cultures. Cell Reports. 2020;**30**:1644-1659. DOI: 10.1016/j.celrep.2020.01.007

[22] Kallman A, Capowski EE, Wang J, Kaushik AM, Jansen AD, Edwards KL, et al. Investigating cone photoreceptor development using patient-derived NRL null retinal organoids. Communications Biology. 2020;**3**:82. DOI: 10.1038/s42003-020-0808-5

[23] Kaewkhaw R, Kaya KD, Brooks M, Homma K, Zou JZ, Chaitankar V, et al. Transcriptome dynamics of developing photoreceptors in three-dimensional retina cultures recapitulates temporal sequence of human cone and rod differentiation revealing cell surface markers and gene networks. Stem Cells. 2015;**33**:3504-3518. DOI: 10.1002/stem.2122

[24] Tao YL, Zhang SC. Neural subtype specification from human pluripotent stem cells. Cell Stem Cell. 2016;**19**:573-586. DOI: 10.1016/j.stem.2016.10.015

[25] Wang Z, Wang SN, Xu TY, Miao ZW, Su DF, Miao CY. Organoid technology for brain and therapeutics research. CNS Neuroscience & Therapeutics. 2017;**23**:771-778. DOI: 10.1111/cns.12754

[26] Cakir B, Xiang YF, Tanaka Y, Kural MH, Parent M, Kang YJ, et al. Engineering of human brain organoids with a functional vascular-like system. Nature Methods. 2019;**16**:1169-1175. DOI: 10.1038/s41592-019-0586-5

[27] Mansour AA, Goncalves JT, Bloyd CW, Li H, Fernandes S, Quang D, et al. An in vivo model of functional and

vascularized human brain organoids. Nature Biotechnology. 2018;**36**:432-441. DOI: 10.1038/nbt.4127

[28] Ao Z, Cai HW, Havert DJ, Wu ZH, Gong ZY, Beggs JM, et al. One-stop microfluidic assembly of human brain organoids to model prenatal cannabis exposure. Analytical Chemistry. 2020;**92**:4630-4638. DOI: 10.1021/acs.analchem.0c00205

[29] Dong X, Xu SB, Chen X, Tao MD, Tang XY, Fang KH, et al. Human cerebral organoids establish subcortical projections in the mouse brain after transplantation. Molecular Psychiatry. 2021;**26**:2964-2976. DOI: 10.1038/s41380-020-00910-4

[30] Kitahara T, Sakaguchi H, Morizane A, Kikuchi T, Miyamoto S, Takahashi J. Axonal extensions along corticospinal tracts from transplanted human cerebral organoids. Stem Cell Reports. 2020;**15**:467-481. DOI: 10.1016/j.stemcr.2020.06.016

[31] Wang Z, Wang SN, Xu TY, Hong C, Cheng MH, Zhu PX, et al. Cerebral organoids transplantation improves neurological motor function in rat brain injury. CNS Neuroscience & Therapeutics. 2020;**26**:682-697. DOI: 10.1111/cns.13286

[32] Wang SN, Wang Z, Xu TY, Cheng MH, Li WL, Miao CY. Cerebral organoids repair ischemic stroke brain injury. Translational Stroke Research. 2020;**11**:983-1000. DOI: 10.1007/s12975-019-00773-0

[33] Nakano T, Ando S, Takata N, Kawada M, Muguruma K, Sekiguchi K, et al. Self-formation of optic cups and storable stratified neural retina from human ESCs. Cell Stem Cell. 2012;**10**:771-785. DOI: 10.1016/j.stem.2012.05.009

[34] Li JY, Chen YJ, Ouyang S, Ma JY, Sun H, Luo LX, et al. Generation and staging of human retinal organoids based on self-formed ectodermal autonomous multi-zone system. Frontiers in Cell and Development Biology. 2021;**9**:732382. DOI: 10.3389/fcell.2021.732382

[35] Wahlin KJ, Maruotti JA, Sripathi SR, Ball J, Angueyra JM, Kim C, et al. Photoreceptor outer segment-like structures in long-term 3D retinas from human pluripotent stem cells. Scientific Reports. 2017;7:766. DOI: 10.1038/s41598-017-00774-9

[36] Souied E, Pulido J, Staurenghi G. Autologous induced stem-cell-derived retinal cells for macular degeneration. The New England Journal of Medicine. 2017;**377**:792. DOI: 10.1056/NEJMc1706274

[37] da Cruz L, Fynes K, Georgiadis O, Kerby J, Luo YH, Ahmado A, et al. Phase 1 clinical study of an embryonic stem cell-derived retinal pigment epithelium patch in age-related macular degeneration. Nature Biotechnology. 2018;**36**:328-337. DOI: 10.1038/nbt.4114

[38] Mehat MS, Sundaram V, Ripamonti C, Robson AG, Smith AJ, Borooah S, et al. Transplantation of human embryonic stem cell-derived retinal pigment epithelial cells in macular degeneration. Ophthalmology. 2018;**125**:1765-1775. DOI: 10.1016/j.ophtha.2018.04.037

[39] Bartsch U, Oriyakhel W, Kenna PF, Linke S, Richard G, Petrowitz B, et al. Retinal cells integrate into the outer nuclear layer and differentiate into mature photoreceptors after subretinal transplantation into adult mice. Experimental Eye Research. 2008;**86**:691-700. DOI: 10.1016/j.exer.2008.01.018

[40] MacLaren RE, Pearson RA, MacNeil A, Douglas RH, Salt TE, Akimoto M, et al. Retinal repair by transplantation of photoreceptor precursors. Nature. 2006;**444**:203-207. DOI: 10.1038/nature05161

[41] Zou T, Gao L, Zeng Y, Li Q, Li Y, Chen S, et al. Organoid-derived C-Kit+/SSEA4- human retinal progenitor cells promote a protective retinal microenvironment during transplantation in rodents. Nature Communications. 2019;**10**:1205. DOI: 10.1038/s41467-019-08961-0

[42] Rabesandratana O, Chaffiol A, Mialot A, Slembrouck-Brec A, Joffrois C, Nanteau C, et al. Generation of a transplantable population of human iPSC-derived retinal ganglion cells. Frontiers in Cell and Development Biology. 2020;**8**:585675. DOI: 10.3389/fcell.2020.585675

[43] Ruzafa N, Vecino E. Effect of Müller cells on the survival and neuritogenesis in retinal ganglion cells. Archivos De La Sociedad Espaola De Oftalmología. 2015;**90**:522-526. DOI: 10.1016/j.oftal.2015.03.009

[44] Gonzalez-Cordero A, Kruczek K, Naeem A, Fernando M, Kloc M, Ribeiro J, et al. Recapitulation of human retinal development from human pluripotent stem cells generates transplantable populations of cone photoreceptors. Stem Cell Reports. 2017;**9**:820-837. DOI: 10.1016/j.stemcr.2017.07.022

[45] Singh MS, Balmer J, Barnard AR, Aslam SA, Moralli D, Green CM, et al. Transplanted photoreceptor precursors transfer proteins to host photoreceptors by a mechanism of cytoplasmic fusion. Nature Communications. 2016;**7**:13537. DOI: 10.1038/ncomms13537

[46] Pearson RA, Gonzalez-Cordero A, West EL, Ribeiro JR, Aghaizu N, Goh D, et al. Donor and host photoreceptors engage in material transfer following transplantation of post-mitotic photoreceptor precursors. Nature Communications. 2016;**7**:13029. DOI: 10.1038/ncomms13029

[47] Schwartz SD, Regillo CD, Lam BL, Eliott D, Rosenfeld PJ, Gregori NZ, et al. Human embryonic stem cell-derived retinal pigment epithelium in patients with age-related macular degeneration and Stargardt's macular dystrophy: Follow-up of two open-label phase 1/2 studies. Lancet. 2015;**385**:509-516. DOI: 10.1016/S0140-6736(14)61376-3

[48] McLelland BT, Lin B, Mathur A, Aramant RB, Thomas BB, Nistor G, et al. Transplanted hESC-derived retina organoid sheets differentiate, integrate, and improve visual function in retinal degenerate rats. Investigative Ophthalmology & Visual Science. 2018;**59**:2586-2603. DOI: 10.1167/iovs.17-23646

[49] Assawachananont J, Mandai M, Okamoto S, Yamada C, Eiraku M, Yonemura S, et al. Transplantation of embryonic and induced pluripotent stem cell-derived 3D retinal sheets into retinal degenerative mice. Stem Cell Reports. 2014;**2**:662-674. DOI: 10.1016/j.stemcr.2014.03.011

[50] Matsuyama T, Tu HY, Sun JA, Hashiguchi T, Akiba R, Sho J, et al. Genetically engineered stem cell-derived retinal grafts for improved retinal reconstruction after transplantation. Iscience. 2021;**24**:102866. DOI: 10.1016/j.isci.2021.102866

[51] Shirai H, Mandai M, Matsushita K, Kuwahara A, Yonemura S, Nakano T, et al. Transplantation of human embryonic stem cell-derived retinal

tissue in two primate models of retinal degeneration. Proceedings of the National Academy of Sciences of the United States of America. 2016;**113**:E81-E90. DOI: 10.1073/pnas.1512590113

[52] Yamasaki S, Tu HY, Matsuyama T, Horiuchi M, Hashiguchi T, Sho J, et al. A Genetic modification that reduces ON-bipolar cells in hESC-derived retinas enhances functional integration after transplantation. iScience. 2021;**25**:103657. DOI: 10.1016/j.isci.2021.103657

[53] Thomas BB, Lin B, Martinez-Camarillo JC, Zhu D, McLelland BT, Nistor G, et al. Co-grafts of human embryonic stem cell derived retina organoids and retinal pigment epithelium for retinal reconstruction in immunodeficient retinal degenerate royal college of surgeons rats. Frontiers in Neuroscience. 2021;**15**:752958. DOI: 10.3389/fnins.2021.752958

[54] Redenti SM, Tao S, Saigal S, Gu P, Yang J, Klassen H, et al. Retinal tissue engineering using mouse retinal progenitor cells and a novel biodegradable poly(e-caprolactone). Nanofiber Scaffold. 2008;**1**:19-29. DOI: 10.1007/s12177-008-9005-3

[55] Yao J, Ko CW, Baranov PY, Regatieri CV, Redenti S, Tucker BA, et al. Enhanced differentiation and delivery of mouse retinal progenitor cells using a micropatterned biodegradable thin-film polycaprolactone scaffold. Tissue Engineering Pt A. 2015;**21**:1247-1260. DOI: 10.1089/ten.TEA.2013.0720

[56] Xian BK, Luo ZM, Li KJ, Li K, Tang MJ, Yang RC, et al. Dexamethasone provides effective immunosuppression for improved survival of retinal organoids after epiretinal transplantation. Stem Cells International. 2019;**2019**:7148032. DOI: 10.1155/2019/7148032

[57] Luo ZM, Xian BK, Li K, Li KJ, Yang RC, Chen MF, et al. Biodegradable scaffolds facilitate epiretinal transplantation of hiPSC-Derived retinal neurons in nonhuman primates. Acta Biomaterialia. 2021;**134**:289-301. DOI: 10.1016/j.actbio.2021.07.040

Chapter 3

The Brain Organoid Technology: Diversity of Protocols and Challenges

Andrey Popatansov

Abstract

The brain organoid technology emerged a little over a decade ago. During this short time span, the handling approach has seen tremendous advancements in order to solve current obstacles and enable the development of new applications. Using these methodologies, the fundamental characteristics of the majority of the brain regions may be mimicked in organoids; however, the existing brain organoids cannot be regarded an exact replica of the human brain or its anatomical regions. This chapter will present some of the biological phenomena on which the brain organoid technology relies. Following this, a summary of the gross common structure and timeline of the brain organoid protocols along with their main components and strategies for their improvement is included. A special selection of protocols for each major brain region will be presented with their origin, rationale, and key specifics. Finally, some of the daunting challenges to brain organoid technology will be highlighted.

Keywords: brain organoids, cerebral organoids, embryoid bodies, methodology, technology, challenges

1. Introduction

More than a decade has passed since the first brain organoid emerged from the lab of one of the fathers of organoid technology – Yoshiki Sasai. During that time, an increasing number of researchers worldwide got attracted by the potential of this technology and the hope that we may learn how to build our brains *in vitro* and thus further adopted and developed it [1]. A few years before the first brain organoid protocol was published, Zhang et al. developed a protocol for the generation of free-floating embryoid bodies (EB) from dissociated human embryonic stem cells (hESC), which afterward could be directed to differentiate into neural precursors in rosette structures. This technique actually was an offspring of the methods for aggregated suspension culture from dissociated fetal brain cells like the one by Bjerkvig et al. from 1986 [2, 3]. The team used cells from post-neurulation stages, when loss of potency is present and which can affect their self-organization and differentiation capacities, as some recent studies reveal, while Zhang et al. used embryonic cells from a much earlier stage of the embryogenesis and therefore could direct them to form neural rosettes (resembling early neural tube-like structures). Noteworthy to mention is the contemporary study by Doetschman et al., in which they could observe nerve cells generated spontaneously and stochastically from EBs formed from blastocyst cells using undefined medium. However, they lacked the knowledge of the molecular mechanisms and ways to direct them to a desired cellular fate [3–6]. Zhang et al. succeeded in generating EBs, which were directed to structures recapitulating very early stages of neural tube formation and comprised mostly of neural precursor cells, thanks to the newer discoveries on the neural induction mechanisms [2]. However, the goal of their study was to get transplantable neural precursors and not to recapitulate later-stage brain regions. Therefore, their protocol was much shorter and more straightforward than the ones for organoids.

By the turn of the twentieth century, the recently acquired knowledge of the molecular control of the embryonic brain patterning got consolidated in updated models of neural induction and morphogenesis. It became evident that the brain morphogenesis is spatiotemporally organized and orchestrated by a dynamic network of transient patterning centers (organizers) that secrete a bunch of molecular controllers (morphogens) that can trigger identity change of nearby cells in a concentration−/distance-dependent fashion. These morphogens are activators or inhibitors of a handful of signaling pathways. In addition, more evidence was accumulated that the neural progenitors without extrinsic signals develop anterior neural specification [7]. So, during the first decade of the new millennium, protocols for stem cell differentiation towards identities from the major brain regions were developed based on this framework. Besides, some of the growth and differentiation conditions were also significantly improved; for example, with the popular dual SMAD inhibition strategy for improved neural induction or with the usage of the survival enhancer of dissociated cells -Y-27632 (ROCK inhibitor that diminishes dissociation-induced apoptosis) [8, 9]. This review will present some of the key biological phenomena engaged in brain organoid generation. The structure and the main components of the brain organoid protocols will be analyzed and summarized. The protocols specific to different brain regions will be presented and analyzed to introduce and guide the readers in this growing field. Furthermore, some of the major obstacles related to brain organoid technology and recapitulating the brain and its regions will be discussed.

2. Brain organoid protocols: general timeline, stages, strategies to improve outcome and classification

Most of the current brain organoid protocols use the dissociation-re-aggregation method to form 3D aggregates from the stem cells. After some period of recovery and establishment of cell–cell contacts and maturation, these aggregates become EBs, which are used as a starting point for organoid formation and development. The EBs are not formed from every stem cell aggregate. So far, the studies have revealed a set of important variables [10, 11]. Firstly, the critical cell mass, i.e., a sufficiently large number of cells, is needed to form EB. Secondly, size and uniformity have a huge effect on the homogeneity and structure of the EBs and may impact the fate choice. Studies found that the addition of Y-27632 is beneficial for these results. To overcome these issues, geometric confinement approaches are often used. Thirdly, the time for aggregation also plays a critical role. These and other variables secure the establishment of an appropriate intra-EB microenvironment to trigger the intrinsic embryo developmental programs. The EBs are multicellular aggregates of stem cells, which resemble the inner cell mass of the pre-gastrulation embryo. These cells have the potential to develop into cells from all three germ layers [12]. Afterward, the cells from the EBs were then committed to neural development through medium change and addition in the medium of various signaling molecules. Initially, during this process of differentiation EBs are directed to neuroectoderm formation. The neuroectoderm then gets transformed to neuroepithelium, which depending on the culturing conditions (as dynamic or static culture) attains the form of large neuroepithelium bulges or small neural rosettes, thus recapitulating the neural tube. These structures further differentiate into more specific brain regions according to the applied patterning scheme [13–16].

The summarized workflow of the procedures and timelines can be divided schematically into the following stages (**Figure 1**), (note that the steps and timeline are exemplary and can vary depending on the organism, used patterning strategies, goals, and other factors) [13–16]:

i. Dissociation of the stem cells and re-aggregation– day −1.

ii. Formation of embryoid bodies – day 0–1. To the embryoid body medium usually is added Y-27632 to increase cell survival. Microscopically the edges of EB have a thin bright ring.

iii. Neural induction – the cells are directed to neuroectodermal fate. Commonly is around 3–6 (10) days for human organoids. The neural induction medium is often supplied with dual SMAD inhibitors (as SB431542 or A83–01 and LDN193189 or dorsomorphin). Microscopically, the edges of EB have a thicker bright ring.

iv. Differentiation – the neuroectoderm is further transformed to neuroepithelium and further expanded. Sometimes this stage is subdivided into two:

v. Region-specific patterning – The differentiation/patterning medium is commonly supplemented with patterning molecules, sometimes also with dual SMAD inhibitors.

vi. Tissue induction and growth – The medium, sometimes, has neural patterning molecules. Often the organoids are embedded or encapsulated in gel in order to prevent the diffusion of the secreted morphogens.

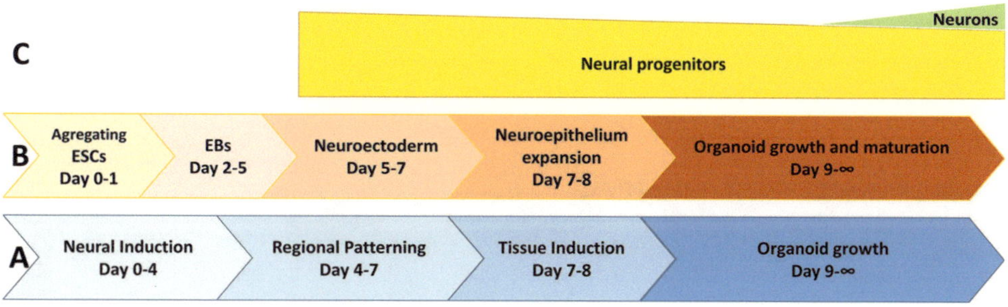

Figure 1.
A schematic timeline of generalized brain organoid protocol: A. stages of the treatments; B. timeline of the 3D culture development and growth; C. timeline of the neural differentiation. After [14–17].

vii. Organoid growth – Maturation medium is commonly used without patterning molecules but instead with growth factors (such as BDNF, NT-3), antioxidants (such as ascorbic acid), and other additives, which enhance the organoid maturation and long-term survival.

Patterning agents: Currently, the available protocols for brain organoids try to mimic the molecular control exercised by the embryonal network of brain patterning centers. The major signaling pathways elaborated or triggered by them are the pathways of fibroblast growth factor (FGF), sonic hedgehog (Shh), Wnt, bone morphogenic protein (BMP), and nodal/activin. This patterning network with its morphogen gradients can be presented in a 3D coordinate system where at each spatial coordinate of the brain primordium corresponds a combination of morphogens (which usually are the first messengers of these pathways) with specific concentrations (**Figure 2**) [19, 20]. Based on this model, the researchers approximate the morphogen combination patterning the region of interest and determine the appropriate concentrations afterward. Although in the brain organoid protocols usually are used as morphogens the first messengers of these pathways, in some scenarios are used secondary messengers or their analogs instead – for example, when it is cost-efficient; or it is difficult to work with them; or is needed partial activation of the pathway or for another reason [21]. In general, the used patterning agents can be divided by their ability to caudalize or ventralize the cell populations regarding the most anterior and dorsal end of the central nervous system primordium. As caudalizing agents, the first messengers from the Wnt and BMP families are often employed, while Shh and Wnt are used as ventralizing agents.

Oxygenation and metabolite exchange: To cope with the lack of vascularization and the hindered oxygen and metabolite exchange, several strategies are developed:

i. Static-to-spinning strategy – during the neural induction and early regional specification phases, the organoids are grown under static conditions and, during the longer stages of growth and maturation, are transferred to a shaker or spinning reactor [22].

ii. Sliced strategy – the growing organoids are regularly sliced during the growth and maturation phase [23].

iii. Air-liquid interface strategy – the maturing organoids, after 2 months are embedded in agarose and cut into slices, one side of which is exposed to air during the consequent culturing [24].

iv. Hyperoxygenation – the air above the brain organoid culture is supplied with extra oxygen (up to 40%) [25].

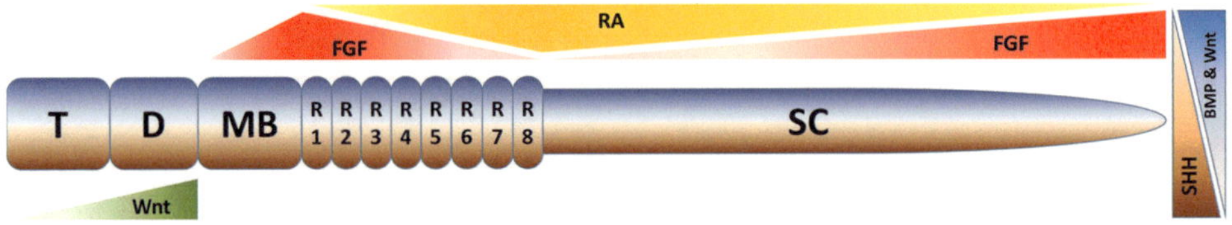

Figure 2.
The morphogen gradients in the developing embryonal CNS. T – Telencephalon; D – Diencephalon; MB – Midbrain; R1-R8 – Rhombomeres of the rhombencephalon; SC – Spinal cord. After [18].

v. Transplantation in animal brain – the maturing organoids are transplanted into the brain of the host animal after one and half months of *in vitro* culture. After a few weeks, the organoids get vascularized and continue to grow in the host [26].

Mediums and Supplements: They are the fundamental components of the organoid microenvironment; however, there is no strict rule on which formulation to use. It requires experimenting with a few recipe/brand choices and their combinations to achieve optimum output. Some commonly used mediums are DMEM/F12; Neurobasal, GlasgowMEM, BrainPhys, mTESR1, Essential medium, etc. [13–16, 27, 28].

As supplements are commonly used: KSR (knockout serum replacement), N2, B27, Gem21 Neuroplex, etc. [13–16, 27, 28].

Stage-dependent medium composition specifics: The biological transformation of the EBs and consequently organoids require adjustment of the microenvironment according to the dynamic transient necessities of the culture. During the initial stages are used DMEM/F12, essential medium supplied with KSR, etc. The medium is often changed during the differentiation stages to Neurobasal, DMEM/F12 with N2, b27(−A). For the maturation stage, often the choice is for Neurobasal, DMEM/F12, or their combination with added supplements [13–17, 27, 28].

Culture dishes and substrates: Dishes with U or V-shaped wells with ultra-low attachment characteristics or hanging drop culture are suggested for the initial stages. At later stages, there is more freedom of dish choice – petri dish, microwells, and microfluidics [13–17, 27, 28]. So far, if a substrate is used at all in the protocols, the most commonly used is Matrigel (basement membrane matrix produced from mouse sarcoma cells); it is used either in differentiation or maturation stages or both [13, 28].

Classification: The current brain organoid protocols can be classified in several ways. One of the commonest is based on the approaches for differentiation and can be divided into two groups: 1. Guided (use external agents to direct the patterning) and 2. Unguided (accentuate on the intrinsic developmental programs) (**Figure 3**) [13–17, 28]. Another way is based on the anatomical region in which the organoids recapitulate – telencephalic, diencephalic, mesencephalic, and rhombencephalic [14–17, 27, 28]. Here will be used in a nested fashion.

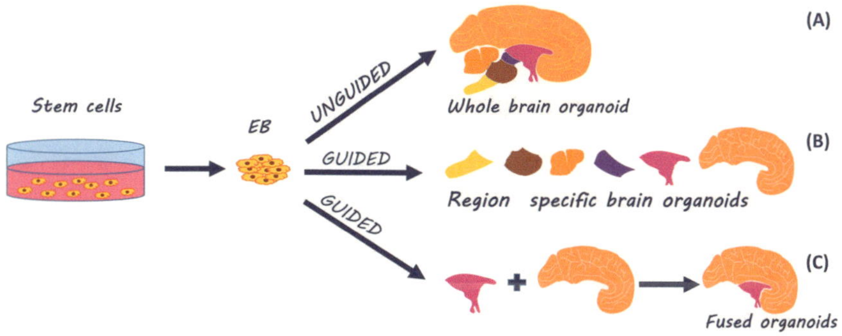

Figure 3.
Approaches for generation of brain organoids. (a). Unguided - without use of patterning agents; (B). And (C). Guided – Utilizing patterning agents to direct the patterning process. (B). Generating region-specific organoids. (C). Generation of fussed organoids from separately grown guided region-specific organoids.

3. Brain organoid protocols – Regional specification

3.1 Guided brain organoids - telencephalon

The telencephalon is the largest part of the brain in humans. Regardless of its astonishing evolutionary expansion in primates, the telencephalon retains its major subdivisions among the vertebrates: 1. The dorsal telencephalon or pallium, which via the thalamus receives most sensory afferents, and 2. Ventral telencephalon subpallium is mainly involved in motor functions (**Figure 4**) [29]. Major organizers are the roof and floor plate and ANR, cortical hem, PSB (pallial-subpallial boundary), or antihem. It may seem that the telencephalon organoids should be the easiest to grow and develop since the default fate of the early embryonic ectodermal cells is one of the rostral telencephalic neurons. However, in reality, this presented a challenge. The first experimental protocols for neural progenitor's induction could derive only neural cells with caudal identity or at best, the midbrain's one [31, 32]. By the early 2000s, an established and empirically discovered neural inducer was the retinoic acid, which induces only neural cells with posterior identity [33].

In the 1990s, few endogenously synthesized molecules were discovered with neural inducing activity, namely Chordin and Follistatin, but they worked for amphibian organisms, while such knowledge was still lacking for the mammalians. One of the leading reasons for this situation was the usage of the animal cap assay as the main workhorse for such discoveries, which is from *Xenopus sp.*, while for mammals, such an assay was missing [32]. Kawasaki et al. in 2000 did an extensive test with a series of perspective molecules for neural induction as FGF2, FGF8, Shh, HGF (hepatocyte growth factor), EGF, PDGF (platelet-derived growth factor), LIF, LiCl (activator of Wnt signaling) on mESC [32, 34]. However, the authors failed to induce neurons with any of them. Instead, they discovered that co-culturing with stromal PA6 cells promotes neural differentiation of mESC, which they named stromal cell-derived inducing activity (SDIA), which seemed to be suppressed by BMP4 treatment (around that time, it was known that BMP4 inhibits neural differentiation [35]. A few years later, Watanabe et al. used a similarly defined medium, but they used SFEB (serum-free

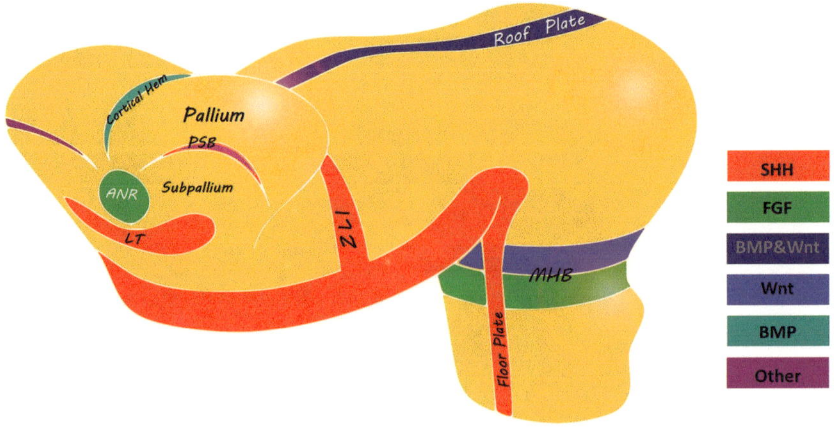

Figure 4.
Organizing centers in the brain primordia with their main morphogens. ANR - anterior neural ridge; ZLI - zona limitans intrathalamica; PSB – Pallial-subpallial boundary; LT - Lamina terminalis; MHB - midbrain-hindbrain boundary. After [29, 30].

floating culture of embryoid body-like aggregates) type culturing instead of attached one [36]. They applied at the beginning during the induction phase Nodal antagonist (LeftyA) since it was found in 2004 that Nodal inhibits ES differentiation to neural fate [37]. In addition, they applied Wnt antagonist (Dkk1), which was in concordance with the neural anteriorizating role of Wnt-inhibitors and caudalizing one of Wnts in the early developmental stages [22]. Later, the authors applied various signaling molecules known to be involved in the brain patterning as Shh and Wnt3a [38, 39].

Eiraku et al. successfully modified the protocol of Watanabe et al. for brain organoids [1, 36]. One of the breakthroughs was shortening the initial aggregation step, which allowed the earlier restoration of the cell–cell interactions. The other facilitating condition was the usage of small bottom micro-well spheroid plates instead of large bottom petri dishes, which improved the aggregation by reducing the number and increasing the size of the formed aggregates. During the late neural induction phase, in the aggregates was formed a cavity through apoptosis similar to those observed by Coucouvanis & Martin in EBs [40]. Thus, forming polarized neuroepithelial structures with an apical surface inside and a basal side outside, which are later divided into smaller neuroepithelial rosettes. Like the mESC culture, the hESC aggregates also formed an internal cavity covered with neuroepithelium; however, they did not reform into smaller rosettes but into mushroom-like shapes. The authors initially applied Dkk1 and LeftyA and later different combinations of FGF8, FGFR3-fc, and BMP4. In this way, they generated polarized tissues recapitulating early corticogenesis of different regions of the forebrain primordium. Few years later, the authors improved this protocol by replacing the partly defined KSR (Knockout Serum Replacement) medium with chemically-defined components [41]. In addition, they added ECM components (as Matrigel, fibronectin, laminin, and laminin/entactin complex) from day 1, which significantly improved the morphological stability of the organoids, especially the later complex. Initially, they applied IWP2 (Wnt inhibitor) and later optionally Shh and FGF8. Thus, they generated cortical neuroepithelium resembling cortical hem-like or lateral ganglionic eminence–like tissues (with Shh addition).

Paşca et al. proposed another approach for generating cortical organoids [42]. Instead of using some of the classical morphogens, they relied on the default neural fate of the ectoderm and the use of some mitogens and growth factors that were found to be able to induce differentiation. Initially, they applied the dual SMAD-inhibition strategy. Afterward, a combination of FGF2 and EGF was applied. Earlier studies have shown the mitogen action of FGF2 and EGF, plus for the EGF, it was found that at later stages, it can also induce differentiation towards neurons and astrocytes [43, 44]. In the next step, the organoids were transferred in a medium with neurotrophic factors BDNF and NT3. As a result, they generated cortical organoids with neurons and astrocytes analogous to the late mid-fetal stage (19–24 weeks post-conception). Next year Qian et al. developed a series of protocols for region-specific organoids [45]. The first type was the forebrain one. They started with a dual SMAD-inhibition strategy (dorsomorphine and A83–01) without morphogens. For the patterning stage, they used CHIR99021, SB431542, and Wnt3a and embedded the organoids in Matrigel. In the next stage, the organoids were detached from the Matrigel and placed in a custom spinning bioreactor. For the maturation stage, growth factors such as BDNF, GDNF, etc., were added. As a result, the authors acquired forebrain organoids with all six cortex layers, which were identified by their respective markers as REELIN, CUX1, BRN2, SATB2, CTIP2, or TBR1.

3.1.1 Guided brain organoids - dorsal telencephalon

The dorsal telencephalon or pallium, for most of its parts, has laminar organization. It can be subdivided into dorsal pallium (isocortex), medial pallium (hippocampus), and lateral pallium (olfactory cortex). The mostly non-neuronal formation of choroid plexus is also included in this region [29, 46]. Kadoshima et al. improved the protocol of Nasu et al. for human dorsal telencephalon organoids [41, 47]. They used the same inhibitors but with tripled cell density. They added FBS and Matrigel in the final step, which improved the long-term growth. In this way, they got organoids of cortical neuroepithelium recapitulating the fetal cortex in the second trimester. Often these organoids formed spontaneously intracortical dorsocaudal-ventrorostral polarity. The neuroepithelium flanking tissue often had cortical hem markers. In a dose-dependent manner with SAG (Shh agonist), they could imitate dorsoventral gradient and generate LGE (lateral ganglionic eminence) and MGE (medial ganglionic eminence) type cells.

Further Mariani et al. optimized the protocol for human-induced pluripotent stem cells (hiPSC) [48]. They used 3-fold higher cell density and Dkk1, SB431542, and BMPRIA-Fc as inhibitors of Wnt, TGF-β/activin/nodal, and BMP pathways. They acquired tissues with a dorsal pallial telencephalic identity corresponding to embryonic human cerebral cortex 8–10 weeks post-conception with stratifying cytoarchitecture, including radial glial cells expressing neural progenitor proteins, intermediate progenitors, and maturing neurons. Later, they used this protocol for patient-specific organoids for autism research [49]. Choroid plexus develops on the dorsal side of the brain ventricles, and its chief functions are the secretion of the cerebrospinal fluid (which has important roles in the homeostasis and neurogenesis) and barrier for the molecular exchange with the vascular system [50]. Therefore, it is the desired target for researchers and medicians alike.

Sakaguchi et al. used the procedure of Kadoshima et al. as a foundation for the production of additional region-specific organoids [51]. At that time, it was known that Wnt and BMP signaling had a leading role in the telencephalon patterning of that region during embryogenesis [52, 53]. First, they explored the ways to generate choroid plexus organoids by using a series of BMPs and a Wnt agonist (CHIR 99021) with different concentrations. As a result, it was found that BMP4 plus CHIR 99021 is the most potent combination, followed by BMP2 and BMP7, and treatment only with CHIR 99021 produces hem-like tissues. The authors also found that the choroid plexus or cortical hem organoids start to produce the patterning ligands characteristic for these organizers in the embryo. Further, they attempted to generate hippocampal primordium tissues. This was achieved by shortening the exposure time to BMP4 plus CHIR 99021, with medium change and additional oxygen supply.

Pellegrini et al. used the protocol for unguided brain organoids of Lancaster et al. to develop a scheme for choroid plexus organoids [13, 54]. The forebrain organoids often have a small percentage of cells with choroid plexus identity. To increase this ratio, an uncommon scheme with pulsed treatment was developed. The authors used the protocols of Watanabe et al. and Sakaguchi et al. to select BMP4 and CHIR 99021 as patterning factors [51, 55]. The generated organoids formed cysts filled with a liquid whose content recapitulates one of the cerebrospinal fluids. Also, the authors found tight barrier formation, the medium and intra-organoid fluid with junction types and transporters characteristic of the native choroid plexus. The marvel of this protocol is that for the first time, such regional organoids could secrete fluid that emulates cerebrospinal fluid and form structures with brain-barrier-like functions.

This provides the researchers with a unique platform to study *in vitro* the mechanisms of the secretion of cerebrospinal fluid or to develop better drugs capable of crossing the blood–brain barrier.

3.1.2 Guided brain organoids - ventral telencephalon

The ventral telencephalon or subpallium has complex and rather dynamic organization and structure during embryogenesis. At E12.5 in mouse, its main subdivisions are: lateral ganglionic eminence (LGE) (produces the striatal components), medial ganglionic eminence (MGE) (pallidum proper and produces globus pallidus), AEP (peduncle/internal capsule, and produces many sublenticular components of the extended amygdala), POC (commissural preoptic area) [56]. So far, specific protocols recapitulating LGE and MGE are developed as described below. Xiang et al. explored the ways to generate brain organoids recapitulating the medial ganglionic eminence [57]. They upgraded the protocol of Maroof et al. for hESC-derived GABAergic interneurons and the one from Nicholas et al. for human pluripotent stem cells (hPSCs)-derived forebrain interneurons [58, 59]. At the neural induction stage, they applied dual SMAD and Wnt inhibitors. For the ventral patterning, they used Shh and purmorphamine. After over 70 days in culture, the MGE organoids comprised diverse cell populations mostly with MGE identity, the largest portion being intermediates or not yet committed, and a quarter were interneurons.

Cederquist et al. applied an unusual approach to generate MGE organoids [60]. They genetically modified a small batch of hPSCs to express sonic hedgehog (Shh) in the presence of doxycycline. Afterward, these cells were dissociated and re-aggregated in small aggregates. On top of them were aggregated 10-fold more hPSCs in this way was created big chimeric spheroid from small Shh producing cell cluster surrounded by a larger mass of non-genetically modified hPSCs. During the neural induction period, dual SMAD and Wnt inhibition and doxycycline were used. In the regional patterning phase, only doxycycline was used. With immunohistochemistry, the authors showed the formation of Shh gradient spreading from the artificial organizer and also that there is regionalization of the organoids recapitulating the dorsoventral patterning of the telencephalon with at least five domains i.e., close to the organizer, the cells had an identity of ventroposterior hypothalamus, next was anterodorsal hypothalamus, then medial ganglionic eminence (MGE) and lateral ganglionic eminence (LGE), and neocortex.

Birey et al. utilized the protocol of Pasca et al. for cortical organoids as the base [42, 61]. In order to get more ventralized organoids, they added IWP-2 (Wnt inhibitor) from the late third of the neural induction stage onwards. And a week later, they added Shh activator (SAG). After 105 days of growth and maturation, the subpallium organoids contained cells with markers for ventral neural progenitors and GABAergic cells. Miura et al. used, as a starting point, the activin-based protocol of Arber et al. for striatal neuron induction in 2D culture to develop a protocol for striatal brain organoids [62, 63]. So, for regional differentiation, initially, they added activin A and IPW2 (Wnt inhibitor). In addition, through transcriptomic analysis, they found that the retinoid X receptor gamma (RXRG) is highly expressed in this region. They added RA agonist (SR11237) and optimized the concentration and time window and found that a week post neural induction phase to be the best time for the agonist application. Afterward, they did a single-cell transcriptomic analysis of the organoids and found that most of the cells were with LGE identity, with over half being GABAergic neurons.

3.2 Guided brain organoids - diencephalon

Diencephalon has still debatable embryonic organization and subdivisions. In mouse at E13.5, it is divided into the hypothalamus, prethalamus, epithalamus, thalamus, and pretectum (**Figure 3**) [64]. Major organizers dorsoventrally are the roof and floor plates and transversely – ZLI (zona limitans intrathalamica). Currently, there are protocols for the hypothalamus, prethalamus, and thalamus as follows.

Shiraishi et al. developed a protocol for stem cell generation of tissues resembling major parts of the diencephalon, and although they did not label them as organoids, it is valuable to be included here [21]. A key component in their rationale was the introduction of the FGF signaling pathway inhibition since FGFs were local caudalizing factors for that region. Their tests showed that the partial intracellular inhibition of MAPK/ERK kinase (MEK) with PD0325901 is better than the total inhibition through the cell membrane FGFR receptor with SU5402. However, these inhibitors brought mediocre gain of cells with thalamic markers. A recent finding by Suzuki-Hirano et al. for strong transient expression of BMP7 in this region helped them to increase the gain significantly by adding BMP7 [65]. Looking further on how to get more differentiated local regionalization, they experimented with activators of Shh (SAG) and Wnt (CHIR 99021) (which are expressed by ZLI). By adding PD0325901 and BMP7 on day 4 and replaced with SAG on day 7, they acquired cell populations from the prethalamus, thalamus (from ventricular and mantle zones), and pretectum in a single sample. When instead SAG was used CHIR99021, it led to an increase of cells with prethalamic markers.

Xiang et al. adapted the protocol of Shiraishi et al. for human forebrain organoids [66]. They changed the Shiraishi et al. timeline and protocol by using dual SMAD inhibition and insulin during the neural induction phase. While for the thalamic patterning phase, they removed them, and it was necessary to inhibit the MEK–ERK signaling (with PD0325901) to prevent excessive caudalization and BMP7 as it promotes thalamic differentiation. They obtained thalamic organoids with strong expression of the thalamic markers TCF7L2 and GBX2. Medina-Cano et al. in order to shorten the time for organoid generation, used epiblast-like cells (EpiLCs) instead of the common blastocyst stem cells [67]. During the first 2 days of neural induction and anterior-posterior patterning phase, they applied dual SMAD along with Wnt and FGF inhibition. For another 2 days during the neuroepithelium expansion, the inhibitors were replaced with FGF8b. From day one till five, the EB were embedded in Matrigel and afterward transferred to an orbital shaker. They found that addition of high levels of FGF8b and no BMP7 (as in [66]) generates organoids with prethalamus identity with higher efficiency.

Ozone et al. improved an adapted for 3D culture previous protocol for 2D hypothalamic cells differentiation [68]. They used twice less KSR supplement for the neural induction medium. While for the patterning phase were, added Shh agonist (SAG) and BMP4. Thus, they gained tissues with the expression of ventral hypothalamic markers. Next protocol developed by Qian et al. was for hypothalamus organoids [45]. They employed dual SMAD inhibition for neural induction. For the specific patterning, they applied Wnt3a, Shh, and purmorphamine. At the differentiation stage, the organoids were transferred to a spinning bioreactor supplied with FGF2 and CTNF (ciliary neurotrophic factor). As a result, the generated organoids after the patterning phase expressed markers for the early hypothalamus development, which later matured to specific hypothalamus cell populations.

3.3 Guided brain organoids - midbrain or mesencephalon

The mesencephalon mainly can be divided (in mouse at E11) into dorsal part - tectum and ventral one - tegmentum. From the ventral midbrain primordium arises substantia nigra, which plays important roles in controlling movement and sensory processing [69, 70]. Its pathology is the key factor in some widespread diseases with a great socio-economic burden as the Parkinson's one [71]. Therefore, significant interest was paid to the midbrain organoids; however, the majority of them are focused on the ventral region (**Figure 4**). Major organizers dorsoventrally are the roof and floor plates and transversely – MHB (midbrain-hindbrain boundary).

Tieng et al. modified 2D culture protocol for midbrain dopaminergic neurons [72, 73]. In the induction phase is used dual SMAD-inhibition plus a cocktail of Shh, purmorphamine (Shh activator), and FGF8 to promote floor plate identity. Shortly, Wnt activator (CHIR99021) is added afterward. The authors also found a positive effect on the maturation by inhibiting Notch pathway, which is known to arrest the proliferation and promote differentiation.

Jo et al. used a slightly different induction and patterning scheme than Tieng et al. by changing the treatment time windows [14]. At the start of the dual SMAD-inhibition, they also added Wnt activator (CHIR99021). On day four were added Shh and FGF8. At the tissue growth phase was added Matrigel and organoids were placed on orbital shaker till the end of the cultivation. In this way, the authors obtained midbrain organoids with neuromelanin-containing and dopamine-secreting neurons. The last protocol developed by Qian et al. was for midbrain organoids and was also based on the 2D protocol for dopaminergic neurons by Kriks et al. [45, 73]. Here, they again used dual SMAD inhibition, but supplied from the beginning with FGF8, Shh and Purmorphamine. Later CHIR99021 was added followed by removal of FGF8, Shh and Purmorphamine and SB431542. Afterwards the organoids were transferred into spinning bioreactors and supplied with growth factors. The obtained midbrain organoids had approx. 50% cells with dopaminergic markers and even more with floor plate identity.

Monzel et al. modified the 2D protocol by Reinhardt et al. for the differentiation of neural precursor cells [74, 75]. Initially, hESC was treated with SB431542, dorsomorphin, CHIR99021, and purmorphamine, and after day four, the first two molecules were removed, and ascorbic acid was added. Thus, after several days, human neuroepithelial stem cells were generated and plated on Matrigel for maintenance. Next, for differentiation into the midbrain, dopaminergic fate CHIR99021 was substituted with FGF8 for 8 days. For the organoid culture, these differentiated cells were dissociated and re-aggregated in the same maintenance medium. On day eight, the aggregates were transferred to Matrigel droplets, and on day 10 were placed long-term in a differentiation medium (with purmorphamine till day 16) on an orbital shaker. After 2 months in culture, the midbrain organoids had over 60% positive midbrain neurons with small percentages of other subtypes and astrocytes.

In an attempt to model Parkinson's disease with midbrain organoids, Smits et al. adapted this protocol by doubling the length of the dual SMAD-inhibition period and afterward reduced 4-fold the concentrations and used SAG instead of purmorphamine in the initial steps [76]. For the differentiation step, FGF8 was used CHIR99021 in static culture. Consequently, Nickels et al. combined these two protocols in order to improve the reproducibility and viability of the organoids [77]. They achieved this by adjusting the initial cell count and changing the timeline of the treatments with respective signaling molecules.

3.4 Guided brain organoids - rhombencephalon or hindbrain

Rhombencephalon is a major part of the 3-vesicle brain primordium in mammals (E9 stage in mouse). In the transition to 5-vesicle brain primordium (E11 in mouse), it divides into two parts - the rostral part metencephalon, which gives rise dorsally to the cerebellum and ventrally to the pons; and the caudal part myelencephalon which gives rise to the medulla oblongata (**Figure 4**) [70]. Major organizers dorsoventrally are the roof and floor plates and transversely - MHB and some rhombomere borders. All main regions were recapitulated by the current hindbrain organoid protocols as described below.

Muguruma et al. upgraded their protocol for 2D culture of cerebellar cells [78, 79]. It would be logical if the authors simply applied some of the morphogens synthesized by the dorsal hindbrain primordia and/or the MHB to direct the cells towards cerebellar identity. However, this approach tried by them, or other researchers led to rather a low efficiency of cerebellar cell generation, especially Purkinje ones [80, 81]. So, they tried somewhat to recapitulate induction of the isthmic organizer, which in turn secretes the needed signaling molecules for cerebellar differentiation. They adapted the strategy of Wataya et al. and used a high dose of the weak caudalizing agent insulin followed by FGF2 (which moderately increased the expression of Wnt1 and FGF8) [78, 82]. Along with that, they applied SB431542, the concentration of which was reduced after a week together with FGF2 [78]. In addition, they found that exogenous FGF19 and SDF1 (stromal-derived factor-1 synthesized by the adjacent meninges) can facilitate cerebellar plate formation.

Brain stem organoids protocol was developed by Eura et al. based on the one from Paşca et al. [42, 83]. Initially, the aggregates were treated with FGF2, EGF, and insulin along with dual-SMAD inhibitors. In addition, they added progesterone and transferrin (engaged in iron metabolism) known to promote dopaminergic differentiation and protection from recent studies [84–86]. On day 22, the used patterning and growth factors were replaced with a cocktail of neurotrophic factors and other small molecules, promoting differentiation and maturation for another week. Afterward, no growth factors were added. In this way, they generated human brainstem organoids (hBSOs), containing midbrain/hindbrain progenitors, noradrenergic and cholinergic neurons, dopaminergic neurons, and neural crest lineage cells. Molchanova et al. developed a protocol for rostral brainstem organoids in a two-step approach [87]. First, they differentiated the stem cells into caudalized human neuroepithelial ones using dual SMAD inhibition along with Wnt and Shh activation. Afterward, the neurospheres were dissociated and re-aggregated to initiate the formation of hindbrain organoids. The caudalized aggregates were treated for a week with Wnt and Shh activators for further differentiation before transfer to the shaker for maturation. After two and 4 months, the organoids had large cell populations with pons and medulla oblongata identity and smaller populations of astrocytes.

Valiulahi et al. used as a starting point the protocol of Kirks et al. for generation of dopamine neurons [73, 88]. Instead of using caudalizing Wnt agonist, they decided to try with the strong caudalizing agent RA. To determine the optimal time window and concentration series of tests were performed and was found that max concentration RA from day one to 13 gives the highest percentage of 5-HT neurons. For the 3D brain organoid protocol, they experimented to find the optimum between RA plus purmorphamine treatment start and the generated structure and set it to day 5 till 13. So, in the end, the dual SMAD inhibitors were omitted in the neural induction phase. Before the end of the patterning phase, the organoids were embedded in Matrigel and later placed on a shaker. As result, they acquired organoids with diverse cell identity which overall resembles the ones from the caudal rhombomeres R5–R8 (which later and the largest population (30–40%) being 5-HT-expressing neurons.

3.5 Unguided brain organoids

Lancaster et al. were the first to develop unguided brain organoids [13]. As a base, they used the protocol of Xia et al. for neuroepithelial differentiation [89]. They added a low concentration of FGF2 and ROCK inhibitor at the initial stage. After 6 days, EB was transferred to a neural induction medium and they began forming neuroepithelial tissues. At the differentiation step, differentiation medium and Matrigel embedding were used. In the final stage, the organoids were transferred to a spinning bioreactor and RA was added. The generated brain organoids were rather large (up to 4 mm) with complex heterogeneous tissues resembling various brain regions such as forebrain, midbrain, and hindbrain.

As you can see the majority of the organoid protocols utilizes only a handful of morphogens and signaling molecules related to the main signaling pathways engaged in the embryonal brain patterning. Among the key points for the success of the protocol is to find the right combination of signaling molecules and their right concentration, the right time and length to apply them. Although most researchers do not publish their error-and-trials reports until they get to the right combination, few do, as Xiang et al. [57, 88], which can be of great help for the newcomer in the field of brain organoids. The quest for better organoids, the demands for cheaper and more reproducible organoids along with other factors in the last few years inspired the researchers to experiment with and introduce some bioengineering approaches in the generation of brain organoids. Howbeit, due to volume limitations here, the reader is encouraged to honor the excellent review by Yi et al. dedicated to the bioengineering approaches in organoids in general [90].

4. Challenges on the path of brain organoids technology

Brain organoid technology is a little over than decade old, and it is still in its infancy. Therefore, it is no surprise that the generated brain organoids still suffer from significant discrepancies compared to the native brain. Here will be discussed some of the important issues.

Vascularization: The brain is one of the most metabolically active organs in the body requiring a high oxygen supply; therefore, it has one of the densest vascularization networks [91, 92]. In most of the current protocols, the brain organoids lack vascularization. Lack of organoid vascularization of such presumably active tissues worsens the viability of the cells, causes necrosis, limits the organoid size, and disturbs the tissue structure [93, 94]. The trouble with the vascularization is mostly due to the fact that the vascular epithelia originate from different germ layers than the neurons and the macroglia [95]. In a recent report, Pham et al. used a dual culture approach by separate differentiation of endothelial cells, which afterward were co-cultured with the formed brain organoids [95]. However, further research is needed to determine how functional the brain organoids are and how well they recapitulate the native brain vascularization. Another proposed approach by Mansour et al. was the implantation of the organoid in the living brain in order to be provoked vascularization from the surrounding tissues, thus securing its long-term survival [96].

Artificial maturation/aging strategies: Currently, most of the organoids develop and differentiate with comparable speed to the one observed during the natural neurogenesis for the particular species [47]. This can be problematic in some applications. For example, if we want to produce an appropriate neural patch for an injured patient using his/her own hiPSC, then this patch generation should happen sufficiently fast in order for the patch to serve its purpose. Alternatively, if we want to study aging-related diseases such as Parkinson's. Borghese et al. used the Notch-inhibition strategy to accelerate the neuronal differentiation of ESC *in vitro* and *in vivo* [97]. However, Notch signaling plays an important role in brain patterning and neuronal specification so that such inhibition may interfere with the desired differentiation results. Miller et al. used progerin (truncated form of lamin, which is associated with premature aging) to induce aging human iPSC [98]. Later Vera et al. proposed another approach by downregulation of telomerase which induces telomere shortening [99]. Recently, Li et al. developed organoids with accelerated growth by using mutant cells; however, such genetically modified organoids cannot be used in translation [100].

Morphological discrepancies with native brain: One of the commonest problems with current brain organoids is that within a single organoid are formed several neuroepithelial rosettes, each acting as a separate center of morphogenesis, while in the normal embryo is formed only one. Recently Knight et al. proposed a protocol for single rosette generation [101]. They achieved a high percentage of single rosette organoids by imposing geometrical confinement on the growth in custom micropatterned plates and/or with ROCK-inhibition.

Glial cells: Most of the brain organoids have little or no glial cells. This is not a big surprise if we consider the gliogenesis timeline during the normal ontogenesis. Significant amounts of astrocytes start to be generated only at the late stages of the embryogenesis, while for the oligodendrocytes, this time starts with the postnatal period [102, 103]. Howbeit, the situation is very different for the microglia, which start to invade the neural tube relatively early in the embryogenesis, and by its end, all the microglia are present [103]. They are absent from the brain organoids because they are produced by different germ layers than the neuroectoderm. So, the lack of glia in the brain organoids is logical, and if we want brain organoids to be better copies of the real brains, then we either need to grow them for a comparable time length of the in vivo brain development or to find shorter ways (for the macroglia) or to introduce somehow the missing germ layer in the system (for the microglia).

There is some recent progress in the resolution of these issues. Ormel et al. modified the unguided protocol of Lancaster et al. by tweaking its timeline and reducing the concentrations of some of the additives, and as a result, they got whole-brain organoids with innate microglial cells [104]. However, this protocol may not be a feasible solution for the researchers who need more specific organoids. Later Bejoy et al. developed a different strategy by dual culturing the brain organoids and the microglia mesodermal progenitors and afterward co-culturing them so that the microglia can invade the organoids [105]. As for the macroglia, Paşca et al. and later Yakoub generated brain organoids that developed together neurons and astrocytes, howbeit they were forebrain specific [42, 106]. Recently Shaker et al. published a protocol for cortical brain organoids that could be used to develop myelinating oligodendrocytes along with astrocytes [107]. All these are encouraging results, so hopefully, we expect to see organoids with full-spectrum glial cells in the future.

5. Concluding remarks

For its short existence, the brain organoid technology made respectable progress and drew lots of interest. It became a rather efficient tool and platform to improve the scientific knowledge of the brain evolution and development and to address clinical problems in a general or personalized approach for brain-related pathologies [13, 45, 48, 49, 108].

Howbeit, there is still large room for improvement and development of this technology since many of its issues wait for practical and efficient solutions and applications.

The functional vascularization of the organoids is probably the most penalizing challenge. When it gets solved, this will open the door for bigger and better replicas of the brain with wider applications as the vascularization network is not only a nutrition/metabolite carrier but also an active part of brain development [109].

Most of the current brain organoids arc rclatively simple mimics of the much more complex brain. For example, at the moment we cannot recapitulate the overwhelming complexity of such a minute brain region as hypothalamus, which is of comparable size to the biggest brain organoids. So far, it is known that tens of signaling molecules dynamically drive the patterning of hypothalamus primordium during early embryogenesis, many of them distributed in a gradient manner with respectable precision [110]. However, the existing hypothalamic brain organoid protocols utilize just two of them in extrinsically uniform concentration. The generated hypothalamic organoids are coarsely differentiated with limited heterogeneity and cell diversity. At later stages, it seems that the control of hypothalamus patterning is also rather complex and poorly known and hard to be recapitulated. Probably better knowledge and experimenting are needed to get an improved recapitulation of this brain region. A promising move in this direction is recent single-cell analysis studies that hold the promise to improve our understanding of the hypothalamus patterning mechanisms [111]. The situation is not very different for the other brain regions than the hypothalamus.

Wider adoption of engineering techniques can help for better and more natural, dynamic control of the microenvironment [90]. They can also improve reproducibility, automate and reduce the costs per organoid.

Another approach to increase the brain organoid complexity is through the fusion of separately grown region-specific ones, thus forming complex structures named assembloids (**Figure 3C**) [112]. Howbeit, this approach is rather young and so far had found limited success and application.

Although the present of the brain organoid technology still seems challenging, looking at the astonishing advances in the embryology and microtechnologies, there is hope that its future could be encouraging with improved products and applications.

Conflict of interest

"The authors declare no conflict of interest."

Author details

Andrey Popatansov
Institute of Neurobiology, Bulgarian Academy of Sciences, Sofia, Bulgaria

*Address all correspondence to: atanasov@abv.bg

References

[1] Eiraku M, Watanabe K, Matsuo-Takasaki M, et al. Self-organized formation of polarized cortical tissues from ESCs and its active manipulation by extrinsic signals. Cell Stem Cell. 2008;**3**(5):519-532. DOI: 10.1016/j.stem.2008.09.002

[2] Zhang SC, Wernig M, Duncan ID, Brüstle O, Thomson JA. In vitro differentiation of transplantable neural precursors from human embryonic stem cells. Nature Biotechnology. 2001;**19**(12):1129-1133. DOI: 10.1038/nbt1201-1129

[3] Bjerkvig R, Steinsvag SK, Laerum OD. Reaggregation of fetal rat brain cells in a stationary culture system. I: Methodology and cell identification. In Vitro Cellular & Developmental Biology. 1986;**22**(4):180-192. DOI: 10.1007/bf02623302

[4] Junyent S, Reeves J, Gentleman E, Habib SJ. Pluripotency state regulates cytoneme selectivity and self-organization of embryonic stem cells. The Journal of Cell Biology. 2021;**220**(4):e202005095. DOI: 10.1083/jcb.202005095

[5] ten Berge D, Koole W, Fuerer C, Fish M, Eroglu E, Nusse R. Wnt signaling mediates self-organization and axis formation in embryoid bodies. Cell Stem Cell. 2008;**3**(5):508-518. DOI: 10.1016/j.stem.2008.09.013

[6] Doetschman TC, Eistetter H, Katz M, Schmidt W, Kemler R. The in vitro development of blastocyst-derived embryonic stem cell lines: Formation of visceral yolk sac, blood islands and myocardium. Journal of Embryology and Experimental Morphology. 1985;**87**:27-45

[7] Gaspard N, Vanderhaeghen P. Mechanisms of neural specification from embryonic stem cells. Current Opinion in Neurobiology. 2010;**20**(1):37-43. DOI: 10.1016/j.conb.2009.12.001

[8] Chambers SM, Fasano CA, Papapetrou EP, Tomishima M, Sadelain M, Studer L. Highly efficient neural conversion of human ES and iPS cells by dual inhibition of SMAD signaling. Nature Biotechnology. 2009;**27**(3):275-280. DOI: 10.1038/nbt.1529

[9] Watanabe K, Ueno M, Kamiya D, et al. A ROCK inhibitor permits survival of dissociated human embryonic stem cells. Nature Biotechnology. 2007;**25**(6):681-686. DOI: 10.1038/nbt1310

[10] Chen KG, Mallon BS, Johnson KR, Hamilton RS, McKay RD, Robey PG. Developmental insights from early mammalian embryos and core signaling pathways that influence human pluripotent cell growth and differentiation. Stem Cell Research. 2014;**12**(3):610-621. DOI: 10.1016/j.scr.2014.02.002

[11] Liyang G, Abdullah S, Rosli R, Nordin N. Neural commitment of embryonic stem cells through the formation of Embryoid bodies (EBs). Malays J Med Sci. 2014;**21**(5):8-16

[12] Weitzer G. Embryonic stem cell-derived embryoid bodies: An in vitro model of eutherian pregastrulation development and early gastrulation. Handbook of Experimental Pharmacology. 2006;**174**:21-51

[13] Lancaster MA, Renner M, Martin CA, et al. Cerebral organoids model human brain development and microcephaly. Nature. 2013;**501**(7467):373-379. DOI: 10.1038/nature12517

[14] Jo J, Xiao Y, Sun AX, et al. Midbrain-like organoids from human pluripotent stem cells contain functional dopaminergic and neuromelanin-producing neurons. Cell Stem Cell. 2016;**19**(2):248-257. DOI: 10.1016/j.stem.2016.07.005

[15] Mohamed NV, Mathur M, da Silva RV, Thomas RA, Lepine P, Beitel LK, et al. Generation of human midbrain organoids from induced pluripotent stem cells. MNI Open Research. 2019;**3**:1. DOI: 10.12688/mniopenres10.12688/mniopenres.12816.2

[16] Sivitilli AA, Gosio JT, Ghoshal B, et al. Robust production of uniform human cerebral organoids from pluripotent stem cells. Life Sci Alliance. 2020;**3**(5):e202000707. DOI: 10.26508/lsa.202000707

[17] Lai JD, Berlind JE, Fricklas G, et al. A model of traumatic brain injury using human iPSC-derived cortical brain organoids. bioRxiv. 2020. 2020.07.05.180299:1-20. DOI: 10.1101/2020.07.05.180299

[18] Brafman D, Willert K. Wnt/β-catenin signaling during early vertebrate neural development. Developmental Neurobiology. 2017;**77**(11):1239-1259. DOI: 10.1002/dneu.22517

[19] Echevarría D, Vieira C, Gimeno L, Martínez S. Neuroepithelial secondary organizers and cell fate specification in the developing brain. Brain Research Reviews. 2003;**43**(2):179-191. DOI: 10.1016/j.brainresrev.2003.08.002

[20] Kiecker C, Lumsden A. Compartments and their boundaries in vertebrate brain development. Nature Reviews. Neuroscience. 2005;**6**(7): 553-564. DOI: 10.1038/nrn1702

[21] Shiraishi A, Muguruma K, Sasai Y. Generation of thalamic neurons from mouse embryonic stem cells. Development. 2017;**144**(7):1211-1220. DOI: 10.1242/dev.144071

[22] Nordström U, Jessell TM, Edlund T. Progressive induction of caudal neural character by graded Wnt signaling. Nature Neuroscience. 2002;**5**(6):525-532. DOI: 10.1038/nn0602-854

[23] Qian X, Su Y, Adam CD, et al. Sliced human cortical Organoids for modeling distinct cortical layer formation. Cell Stem Cell. 2020;**26**(5):766-781.e9. DOI: 10.1016/j.stem.2020.02.002

[24] Giandomenico SL, Mierau SB, Gibbons GM, et al. Cerebral organoids at the air-liquid interface generate diverse nerve tracts with functional output. Nature Neuroscience. 2019;**22**(4):669-679. DOI: 10.1038/s41593-019-0350-2

[25] Watanabe M, Buth JE, Vishlaghi N, et al. Self-organized cerebral Organoids with human-specific features predict effective drugs to combat Zika virus infection. Cell Reports. 2017;**21**(2):517-532. DOI: 10.1016/j.celrep.2017.09.047

[26] Daviaud N, Friedel RH, Zou H. Vascularization and engraftment of transplanted human cerebral Organoids in mouse cortex. eNeuro. 2018;**5**(6):219-218. DOI: 10.1523/ENEURO.0219-18.2018

[27] Lin Y, Chen G. Embryoid body formation from human pluripotent stem cells in chemically defined E8 media. In: Stem Book. Cambridge (MA): Harvard Stem Cell Institute; 2008. DOI: 10.3824/stembook.1.98.1

[28] Tanaka Y, Cakir B, Xiang Y, Sullivan GJ, Park IH. Synthetic analyses of single-cell Transcriptomes from multiple brain Organoids and fetal brain. Cell Reports. 2020;**30**(6):1682-1689.e3. DOI: 10.1016/j.celrep.2020.01.038

[29] Montiel JF, Aboitiz F. Pallial patterning and the origin of the isocortex.

Frontiers in Neuroscience. 2015;**9**:377. DOI: 10.3389/fnins.2015.00377

[30] Kiecker C, Lumsden A. The role of organizers in patterning the nervous system. Annual Review of Neuroscience. 2012;**35**(1):347-367. DOI: 10.1146/annurev-neuro-062111-150543

[31] Bain G, Kitchens D, Yao M, Huettner JE, Gottlieb DI. Embryonic stem cells express neuronal properties in vitro. Developmental Biology. 1995;**168**(2):342-357. DOI: 10.1006/dbio.1995.1085

[32] Kawasaki H, Mizuseki K, Nishikawa S, et al. Induction of midbrain dopaminergic neurons from ES cells by stromal cell-derived inducing activity. Neuron. 2000;**28**(1):31-40. DOI: 10.1016/s0896-6273(00)00083-0

[33] Bain G, Ray WJ, Yao M, Gottlieb DI. Retinoic acid promotes neural and represses mesodermal gene expression in mouse embryonic stem cells in culture. Biochemical and Biophysical Research Communications. 1996;**223**(3):691-694. DOI: 10.1006/bbrc.1996.0957

[34] Hedgepeth CM, Conrad LJ, Zhang J, Huang HC, Lee VM, Klein PS. Activation of the Wnt signaling pathway: A molecular mechanism for lithium action. Developmental Biology. 1997;**185**(1):82-91. DOI: 10.1006/dbio.1997.8552

[35] Finley MF, Devata S, Huettner JE. BMP-4 inhibits neural differentiation of murine embryonic stem cells. Journal of Neurobiology. 1999;**40**(3):271-287. DOI: 10.1002/(sici)1097-4695(19990905)40:3<271::aid-neu1>3.0.co;2-c

[36] Watanabe K, Kamiya D, Nishiyama A, et al. Directed differentiation of telencephalic precursors from embryonic stem cells. Nature Neuroscience. 2005;**8**(3):288-296. DOI: 10.1038/nn1402

[37] Vallier L, Reynolds D, Pedersen RA. Nodal inhibits differentiation of human embryonic stem cells along the neuroectodermal default pathway. Developmental Biology. 2004;**275**(2):403-421. DOI: 10.1016/j.ydbio.2004.08.031

[38] Ericson J, Muhr J, Placzek M, Lints T, Jessell TM, Edlund T. Sonic hedgehog induces the differentiation of ventral forebrain neurons: A common signal for ventral patterning within the neural tube. Cell. 1995;**81**(5):747-756. DOI: 10.1016/0092-8674(95)90536-7

[39] Lee SM, Tole S, Grove E, McMahon AP. A local Wnt-3a signal is required for development of the mammalian hippocampus. Development. 2000;**127**(3):457-467. DOI: 10.1242/dev.127.3.457

[40] Coucouvanis E, Martin GR. Signals for death and survival: A two-step mechanism for cavitation in the vertebrate embryo. Cell. 1995;**83**(2):279-287. DOI: 10.1016/0092-8674(95)90169-8

[41] Nasu M, Takata N, Danjo T, et al. Robust formation and maintenance of continuous stratified cortical neuroepithelium by laminin-containing matrix in mouse ES cell culture. PLoS One. 2012;**7**(12):e53024. DOI: 10.1371/journal.pone.0053024

[42] Paşca AM, Sloan SA, Clarke LE, et al. Functional cortical neurons and astrocytes from human pluripotent stem cells in 3D culture. Nature Methods. 2015;**12**(7):671-678. DOI: 10.1038/nmeth.3415

[43] Gensburger C, Labourdette G, Sensenbrenner M. Brain basic fibroblast growth factor stimulates the proliferation

of rat neuronal precursor cells in vitro. FEBS Letters. 1987;**217**(1):1-5. DOI: 10.1016/0014-5793(87)81230-9

[44] Reynolds BA, Tetzlaff W, Weiss S. A multipotent EGF-responsive striatal embryonic progenitor cell produces neurons and astrocytes. The Journal of Neuroscience. 1992;**12**(11):4565-4574. DOI: 10.1523/jneurosci.12-11-04565.1992

[45] Qian X, Nguyen HN, Song MM, et al. Brain-region-specific organoids using mini-bioreactors for modeling ZIKV exposure. Cell. 2016;**165**(5):1238-1254. DOI: 10.1016/j.cell.2016.04.032

[46] Lun MP, Monuki ES, Lehtinen MK. Development and functions of the choroid plexus-cerebrospinal fluid system. Nature Reviews. Neuroscience. 2015;**16**(8):445-457. DOI: 10.1038/nrn3921

[47] Kadoshima T, Sakaguchi H, Nakano T, et al. Self-organization of axial polarity, inside-out layer pattern, and species-specific progenitor dynamics in human ES cell-derived neocortex. Proceedings of the National Academy of Sciences of the United States of America. 2013;**110**(50):20284-20289. DOI: 10.1073/pnas.1315710110

[48] Mariani J, Simonini MV, Palejev D, et al. Modeling human cortical development in vitro using induced pluripotent stem cells. Proc Natl Acad Sci USA. 2012;**109**(31):12770-12775. DOI: 10.1073/pnas.1202944109

[49] Mariani J, Coppola G, Zhang P, et al. FOXG1-dependent dysregulation of GABA/glutamate neuron differentiation in autism spectrum disorders. Cell. 2015;**162**(2):375-390. DOI: 10.1016/j.cell.2015.06.034

[50] Johansson PA. The choroid plexuses and their impact on developmental neurogenesis. Frontiers in Neuroscience. 2014;**8**:340. DOI: 10.3389/fnins.2014.00340

[51] Sakaguchi H, Kadoshima T, Soen M, et al. Generation of functional hippocampal neurons from self-organizing human embryonic stem cell-derived dorsomedial telencephalic tissue. Nature Communications. 2015;**6**(1):8896. DOI: 10.1038/ncomms9896

[52] Furuta Y, Piston DW, Hogan BL. Bone morphogenetic proteins (BMPs) as regulators of dorsal forebrain development. Development. 1997;**124**(11):2203-2212. DOI: 10.1242/dev.124.11.2203

[53] Grove EA, Tole S, Limon J, Yip L, Ragsdale CW. The hem of the embryonic cerebral cortex is defined by the expression of multiple Wnt genes and is compromised in Gli3-deficient mice. Development. 1998;**125**(12):2315-2325. DOI: 10.1242/dev.125.12.2315

[54] Pellegrini L, Bonfio C, Chadwick J, Begum F, Skehel M, Lancaster MA. Human CNS barrier-forming organoids with cerebrospinal fluid production. Science. 2020;**369**(6500):eaaz5626. DOI: 10.1126/science.aaz5626

[55] Watanabe M, Kang YJ, Davies LM, et al. BMP4 sufficiency to induce choroid plexus epithelial fate from embryonic stem cell-derived neuroepithelial progenitors. The Journal of Neuroscience. 2012;**32**(45):15934-15945. DOI: 10.1523/JNEUROSCI.3227-12.2012

[56] García-López M, Abellán A, Legaz I, Rubenstein JL, Puelles L, Medina L. Histogenetic compartments of the mouse centromedial and extended amygdala based on gene expression patterns during development. The Journal of Comparative Neurology. 2008;**506**(1):46-74. DOI: 10.1002/cne.21524

[57] Xiang Y, Tanaka Y, Patterson B, et al. Fusion of regionally specified hPSC-derived organoids models human brain development and interneuron migration. Cell Stem Cell. 2017;**21**(3):383-398.e7. DOI: 10.1016/j.stem.2017.07.007

[58] Maroof AM, Keros S, Tyson JA, et al. Directed differentiation and functional maturation of cortical interneurons from human embryonic stem cells. Cell Stem Cell. 2013;**12**(5):559-572. DOI: 10.1016/j.stem.2013.04.008

[59] Nicholas CR, Chen J, Tang Y, et al. Functional maturation of hPSC-derived forebrain interneurons requires an extended timeline and mimics human neural development. Cell Stem Cell. 2013;**12**(5):573-586. DOI: 10.1016/j.stem.2013.04.005

[60] Cederquist GY, Asciolla JJ, Tchieu J, et al. Specification of positional identity in forebrain organoids. Nature Biotechnology. 2019;**37**(4):436-444. DOI: 10.1038/s41587-019-0085-3

[61] Birey F, Andersen J, Makinson CD, et al. Assembly of functionally integrated human forebrain spheroids. Nature. 2017;**545**(7652):54-59. DOI: 10.1038/nature22330

[62] Arber C, Precious SV, Cambray S, et al. Activin a directs striatal projection neuron differentiation of human pluripotent stem cells. Development. 2015;**142**(7):1375-1386. DOI: 10.1242/dev.117093

[63] Miura Y, Li MY, Birey F, et al. Generation of human striatal organoids and cortico-striatal assembloids from human pluripotent stem cells. Nature Biotechnology. 2020;**38**(12):1421-1430. DOI: 10.1038/s41587-020-00763-w

[64] Puelles L, Martinez S. Patterning of the diencephalon. In: Patterning and Cell Type Specification in the Developing CNS and PNS. Amsterdam: Elsevier; 2013. pp. 151-172. DOI: 10.1016/b978-0-12-397265-1.00048-4

[65] Suzuki-Hirano A, Ogawa M, Kataoka A, et al. Dynamic spatiotemporal gene expression in embryonic mouse thalamus. The Journal of Comparative Neurology. 2011;**519**(3):528-543. DOI: 10.1002/cne.22531

[66] Xiang Y, Tanaka Y, Cakir B, et al. HESC-derived thalamic organoids form reciprocal projections when fused with cortical organoids. Cell Stem Cell. 2019;**24**(3):487-497.e7. DOI: 10.1016/j.stem.2018.12.015

[67] Medina-Cano D, Corrigan EK, Glenn R, et al. Rapid and robust directed differentiation of mouse epiblast stem cells into definitive endoderm and forebrain organoids. bioRxiv. 2021. 2021.12.07.471652:1-37. DOI: 10.1101/2021.12.07.471652

[68] Ozone C, Suga H, Eiraku M, et al. Functional anterior pituitary generated in self-organizing culture of human embryonic stem cells. Nature Communications. 2016;7(1):10351. DOI: 10.1038/ncomms10351

[69] Prakash N, Wurst W. Specification of midbrain territory. Cell and Tissue Research. 2004;**318**(1):5-14. DOI: 10.1007/s00441-004-0955-x

[70] Chen VS, Morrison JP, Southwell MF, Foley JF, Bolon B, Elmore SA. Histology atlas of the developing prenatal and postnatal mouse central nervous system, with emphasis on prenatal days E7.5 to E18.5. Toxicologic Pathology. 2017;**45**(6):705-744. DOI: 10.1177/0192623317728134

[71] Delenclos M, Jones DR, McLean PJ, Uitti RJ. Biomarkers in Parkinson's

disease: Advances and strategies. Parkinsonism & Related Disorders. 2016;**22**(Suppl. 1):S106-S110. DOI: 10.1016/j.parkreldis.2015.09.048

[72] Tieng V, Stoppini L, Villy S, Fathi M, Dubois-Dauphin M, Krause KH. Engineering of midbrain organoids containing long-lived dopaminergic neurons. Stem Cells and Development. 2014;**23**(13):1535-1547. DOI: 10.1089/scd.2013.0442

[73] Kriks S, Shim JW, Piao J, et al. Dopamine neurons derived from human ES cells efficiently engraft in animal models of Parkinson's disease. Nature. 2011;**480**(7378):547-551. DOI: 10.1038/nature10648

[74] Monzel AS, Smits LM, Hemmer K, et al. Derivation of human midbrain-specific organoids from neuroepithelial stem cells. Stem Cell Reports. 2017;**8**(5):1144-1154. DOI: 10.1016/j.stemcr.2017.03.010

[75] Reinhardt P, Glatza M, Hemmer K, et al. Derivation and expansion using only small molecules of human neural progenitors for neurodegenerative disease modeling. PLoS One. 2013;**8**(3):e59252. DOI: 10.1371/journal.pone.0059252

[76] Smits LM, Reinhardt L, Reinhardt P, et al. Modeling Parkinson's disease in midbrain-like organoids. NPJ Parkinsons Dis. 2019;**5**(1):5. DOI: 10.1038/s41531-019-0078-4

[77] Nickels SL, Modamio J, Mendes-Pinheiro B, Monzel AS, Betsou F, Schwamborn JC. Reproducible generation of human midbrain organoids for in vitro modeling of Parkinson's disease. Stem Cell Research. 2020;**46**(101870):101870. DOI: 10.1016/j.scr.2020.101870

[78] Muguruma K, Nishiyama A, Kawakami H, Hashimoto K, Sasai Y. Self-organization of polarized cerebellar tissue in 3D culture of human pluripotent stem cells. Cell Reports. 2015;**10**(4):537-550. DOI: 10.1016/j.celrep.2014.12.051

[79] Muguruma K, Nishiyama A, Ono Y, et al. Ontogeny-recapitulating generation and tissue integration of ES cell-derived Purkinje cells. Nature Neuroscience. 2010;**13**(10):1171-1180. DOI: 10.1038/nn.2638

[80] Su HL, Muguruma K, Matsuo-Takasaki M, Kengaku M, Watanabe K, Sasai Y. Generation of cerebellar neuron precursors from embryonic stem cells. Developmental Biology. 2006;**290**(2):287-296. DOI: 10.1016/j.ydbio.2005.11.010

[81] Salero E, Hatten ME. Differentiation of ES cells into cerebellar neurons. Proceedings of the National Academy of Sciences of the United States of America. 2007;**104**(8):2997-3002. DOI: 10.1073/pnas.0610879104

[82] Wataya T, Ando S, Muguruma K, et al. Minimization of exogenous signals in ES cell culture induces rostral hypothalamic differentiation. Proceedings of the National Academy of Sciences of the United States of America. 2008;**105**(33):11796-11801. DOI: 10.1073/pnas.0803078105

[83] Eura N, Matsui TK, Luginbühl J, et al. Brainstem organoids from human pluripotent stem cells. Frontiers in Neuroscience. 2020;**14**:538. DOI: 10.3389/fnins.2020.00538

[84] Díaz NF, Díaz-Martínez NE, Velasco I, Camacho-Arroyo I. Progesterone increases dopamine neurone number in differentiating mouse embryonic stem cells. Journal of Neuroendocrinology. 2009;**21**(8):730-736. DOI: 10.1111/j.1365-2826.2009.01891.x

[85] Ayton S, Lei P, Mclean C, Bush AI, Finkelstein DI. Transferrin protects against Parkinsonian neurotoxicity and is deficient in Parkinson's substantia nigra. Signal Transduction and Targeted Therapy. 2016;**1**:16015. DOI: 10.1038/sigtrans.2016.15

[86] Lee JE, Lim MS, Park JH, Park CH, Koh HC. PTEN promotes dopaminergic neuronal differentiation through regulation of ERK-dependent inhibition of S6K signaling in human neural stem cells. Stem Cells Translational Medicine. 2016;**5**(10):1319-1329. DOI: 10.5966/sctm.2015-0200

[87] Molchanova SM, Cherepkova MY, Abdurakhmanova S, et al. Maturation of neuronal activity in Caudalized human brain Organoids. bioRxiv. 2019. 779355:1-45. DOI: 10.1101/779355

[88] Valiulahi P, Vidyawan V, Puspita L, et al. Generation of caudal-type serotonin neurons and hindbrain-fate organoids from hPSCs. Stem Cell Reports. 2021;**16**(8):1938-1952. DOI: 10.1016/j.stemcr.2021.06.006

[89] Xia X, Zhang SC. Differentiation of neuroepithelia from human embryonic stem cells. Methods in Molecular Biology. 2009;**549**:51-58. DOI: 10.1007/978-1-60327-931-4_4

[90] Yi SA, Zhang Y, Rathnam C, Pongkulapa T, Lee KB. Bioengineering approaches for the advanced organoid research. Advanced Materials. 2021;**33**(45):e2007949. DOI: 10.1002/adma.202007949

[91] Watts ME, Pocock R, Claudianos C. Brain energy and oxygen metabolism: Emerging role in normal function and disease. Frontiers in Molecular Neuroscience. 2018;**11**:216. DOI: 10.3389/fnmol.2018.00216

[92] Bohn KA, Adkins CE, Mittapalli RK, et al. Semi-automated rapid quantification of brain vessel density utilizing fluorescent microscopy. Journal of Neuroscience Methods. 2016;**270**:124-131. DOI: 10.1016/j.jneumeth.2016.06.012

[93] Shen Q, Goderie SK, Jin L, et al. Endothelial cells stimulate self-renewal and expand neurogenesis of neural stem cells. Science. 2004;**304**(5675):1338-1340. DOI: 10.1126/science.1095505

[94] Yin X, Mead BE, Safaee H, Langer R, Karp JM, Levy O. Engineering stem cell organoids. Cell Stem Cell. 2016;**18**(1):25-38. DOI: 10.1016/j.stem.2015.12.005

[95] Pham MT, Pollock KM, Rose MD, et al. Generation of human vascularized brain organoids. Neuroreport. 2018;**29**(7):588-593. DOI: 10.1097/WNR.0000000000001014

[96] Mansour AA, Gonçalves JT, Bloyd CW, et al. An in vivo model of functional and vascularized human brain organoids. Nature Biotechnology. 2018;**36**(5):432-441. DOI: 10.1038/nbt.4127

[97] Borghese L, Dolezalova D, Opitz T, et al. Inhibition of notch signaling in human embryonic stem cell-derived neural stem cells delays G1/S phase transition and accelerates neuronal differentiation in vitro and in vivo. Stem Cells. 2010;**28**(5):955-964. DOI: 10.1002/stem.408

[98] Miller JD, Ganat YM, Kishinevsky S, et al. Human iPSC-based modeling of late-onset disease via progerin-induced aging. Cell Stem Cell. 2013;**13**(6):691-705. DOI: 10.1016/j.stem.2013.11.006

[99] Vera E, Bosco N, Studer L. Generating late-onset human iPSC-based disease models by inducing neuronal age-related phenotypes through

telomerase manipulation. Cell Reports. 2016;**17**(4):1184-1192. DOI: 10.1016/j.celrep.2016.09.062

[100] Li Y, Muffat J, Omer A, et al. Induction of expansion and folding in human cerebral organoids. Cell Stem Cell. 2017;**20**(3):385-396.e3. DOI: 10.1016/j.stem.2016.11.017

[101] Knight GT, Lundin BF, Iyer N, et al. Engineering induction of singular neural rosette emergence within hPSC-derived tissues. eLife. 2018;7:e37549. DOI: 10.7554/eLife.37549

[102] Chandrasekaran A, Avci HX, Leist M, Kobolák J, Dinnyés A. Astrocyte differentiation of human pluripotent stem cells: New tools for neurological disorder research. Frontiers in Cellular Neuroscience. 2016;**10**:215. DOI: 10.3389/fncel.2016.00215

[103] Reemst K, Noctor SC, Lucassen PJ, Hol EM. The indispensable roles of microglia and astrocytes during brain development. Frontiers in Human Neuroscience. 2016;**10**:566. DOI: 10.3389/fnhum.2016.00566

[104] Ormel PR, Vieira R, Bodegraven EJ, et al. Microglia innately develop within cerebral organoids. Nature Communications. 2018;**9**(1):4167. DOI: 10.1038/s41467-018-06684-2

[105] Bejoy J, Yuan X, Song L, et al. Genomics analysis of metabolic pathways of human stem cell-derived microglia-like cells and the integrated cortical spheroids. Stem Cells International. 2019;**2019**:2382534. DOI: 10.1155/2019/2382534

[106] Yakoub AM. Cerebral organoids exhibit mature neurons and astrocytes and recapitulate electrophysiological activity of the human brain. Neural Regeneration Research. 2019;**14**(5):757-761. DOI: 10.4103/1673-5374.249283

[107] Shaker MR, Pietrogrande G, Martin S, Lee JH, Sun W, Wolvetang EJ. Rapid and efficient generation of myelinating human oligodendrocytes in organoids. Frontiers in Cellular Neuroscience. 2021;**15**:631548. DOI: 10.3389/fncel.2021.631548

[108] Cárdenas A, Villalba A, de Juan RC, et al. Evolution of cortical neurogenesis in amniotes controlled by Robo signaling levels. Cell. 2018;**174**(3):590-606.e21. DOI: 10.1016/j.cell.2018.06.007

[109] Tata M, Ruhrberg C. Cross-talk between blood vessels and neural progenitors in the developing brain. Neuronal. Signals. 2018;**2**(1):NS20170139. DOI: 10.1042/NS20170139

[110] Bedont JL, Newman EA, Blackshaw S. Patterning, specification, and differentiation in the developing hypothalamus. Wiley Interdisciplinary Reviews: Developmental Biology. 2015;**4**(5):445-468. DOI: 10.1002/wdev.187

[111] Romanov RA, Tretiakov EO, Kastriti ME, et al. Molecular design of hypothalamus development. Nature. 2020;**582**(7811):246-252. DOI: 10.1038/s41586-020-2266-0

[112] Paşca SP. Assembling human brain organoids. Science. 2019;**363**(6423):126-127. DOI: 10.1126/science.aau5729

Section 3

Retinal Organoid

Chapter 4

Retinal Organoids over the Decade

Jing Yuan and Zi-Bing Jin

Abstract

Retinal organoids (ROs) are 3D tissue structures derived from embryonic stem cells (ESCs) or induced pluripotent stem cells (iPSCs) in vitro, which characterize the structure and function of retina to a certain extent. Since 2011, mouse and human retinal organoids have been available, opening up new avenues for retinal development, disease and regeneration research. Over the decade, great progress has been made in the development of retinal organoids, which is reflected in the improvement of differentiation efficiency and development degree. At the same time, retinal organoids also show broad application prospects, which are widely used in the construction of disease models. On this basis, the mechanism of disease, drug screening and retinal regeneration therapy have been explored. Although retinal organoids have a bright future, the deficiency of their structure and function, the limitations of differentiation and culture, and the difference compared with embryonic retina still remain to be solved.

Keywords: retinal organoids, retinal differentiation, disease models, retinal degenerative diseases, transplant

1. Introduction

Located in the back of eyeball, the retina is a soft and transparent membrane attached to the inner surface of the choroid and forms part of the central nervous system. The retina can sense light stimuli, convert the light signals it receives into electrical signals, and then transmit them to the cerebral cortex through the optic nerve to form vision [1]. The retina is mainly composed of pigment epithelial cells, photoreceptor cells, bipolar cells, horizontal cells, amacrine cells, ganglion cells, and Müller glial cells [2]. Different neuron types form different layers, and the orderly arranged nuclei and synaptic regions are alternately arranged, forming a complex and orderly layered structure of the retina [3].

Our early research on the retina, derived only from human fetal retinal tissue [4, 5], faced significant challenges due to access difficulties and ethical issues [6]. Beyond that, most of what we know about the retina comes from studying animal retinas, but human and animal retinas differ in composition and function. For example, most mammals have only two types of cone photoreceptors that express S-opsin or M-opsin [7, 8], while humans have a third type that expresses L-opsin [9]; mice, the main subjects of our study, have a higher proportion of rods than humans [10], whose vision is determined by the density of cones in the macula and fovea [11, 12]. Therefore, it is of great significance to develop appropriate human retinal models to supplement animal models.

The establishment of human embryonic stem cell (ESC) lines [13] and the emergence of induced pluripotent stem cell (iPSC) technology [14] have turned our attention to cell research. Early 2D differentiation protocols used exogenous signaling molecules, Wnt antagonist DKK1 and bone morphogenetic protein (BMP) antagonist Noggin, to guide pluripotent stem cells to an anterior neural fate [15–17] and to differentiate into various types of retinal cells, including retinal pigment epithelial (RPE) cells, photoreceptors, and ganglion cells [18–25]. However, 2D differentiation is far from interpreting retinal development in vivo. Retinal development and maturation are regulated by a series of interacting signal networks, such as factors secreted by RPE that promote photoreceptor maturation. Early retinal differentiation produced a single cell type [19–22] and lacked the necessary interaction between cells. Therefore, we still need to find a more perfect model of human retina.

This breakthrough was achieved by constructing a 3D differentiation procedure. Through 3D differentiation, we can obtain retinal organoids that are highly reducible to the development process and complex structure of the retina, which we vividly call it "retina in a dish." In this chapter, we review the development of retinal organoids and show their application in today's life science research.

2. Overview of retinal organoids

In 2011, Sassi's team used mouse embryonic stem cells (mESCs) to construct the first true retinal organoid through a 3D differentiation procedure [26]. In the following year, human retinal organoids were created [27], which is of epoch-making significance, meaning that human research on retinal development and retinal diseases has entered a new stage, and retinal organoids also provide a new and most potential tool for the treatment of retinal degeneration diseases.

During neurogenesis in vertebrates, the development of the retina can be roughly divided into two stages, the appearance of the optic cup structure and the orderly differentiation of seven types of retinal cells. In the first stage, the forebrain splits to form two secondary brain vesicles: telencephalon and diencephalon. In the diencephalon, eye field region first bulges outward to form the optic vesicle, and the distal vesicle invaginates to form the double-layer optic cup, which further develops into the outer retinal pigment epithelium and the inner neural retina (NR) (**Figure 1a**) [28–32]. In the second stage, the inner pluripotent retinal progenitor cells (RPCs) sequentially differentiate into retinal ganglion cells (RGCs), cone photoreceptors, horizontal cells, amacrine cells, rod photoreceptors, bipolar cells and Müller glia cells (**Figure 1b**) [33]. The cone and rod are connected to the retinal pigment epithelium and together form the outer nuclear layer (ONL). After extending to the outer plexiform layer (OPL), they form synapses with bipolar cells and horizontal cells in the inner nuclear layer (INL). On the other side of the inner nuclear layer, bipolar cells, amacrine cells, and ganglion cells form the synaptic networks of the inner plexiform layer (IPL). Müller glial cells span the whole layer of the retina, from the retinal pigment epithelium to the ganglion cell layer (GCL) (**Figure 1c**) [34, 35].

Retinal development in vivo is regulated by a series of transcription factors, signal transduction factors and cell surface factors. In vitro, differentiation of retinal organoids is also a programmed process that mimics development in vivo by adding various signaling molecules in stages. First, stem cells proliferate and aggregate (**Figure 2A**), inducing the formation of embryoid body (EB) (**Figure 2B**) and neuroepithelium (**Figure 2C**), which appear as translucent bright rings under a microscope (**Figure 2D**). And then,

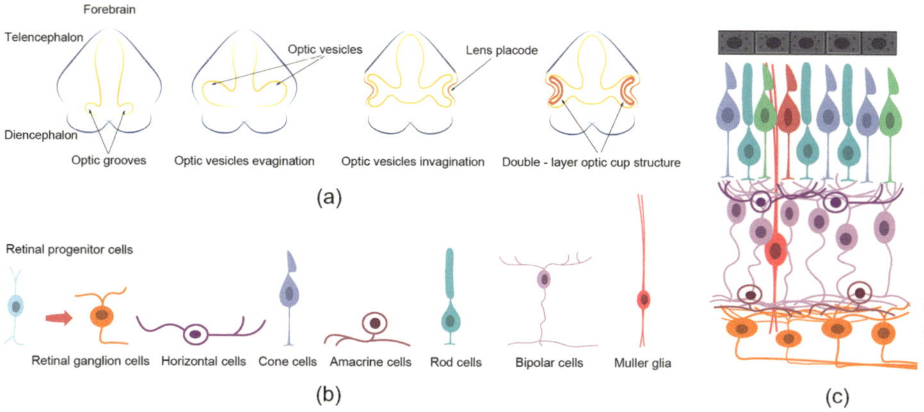

Figure 1.
Overview of retina. (a) the first stage of retinal development: The formation of double—Layer optic cup structure. (b) the second stage of retinal development: Retinal progenitor cells (RPCs) differentiate into seven types of retinal cells. (c) Structure of the retina.

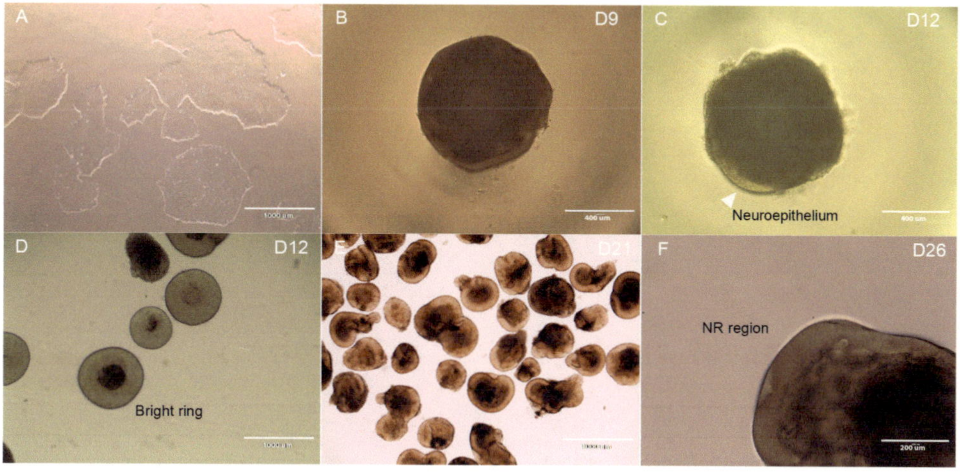

Figure 2.
The differentiation of retinal organoids. (A) Growing human embryonic stem cells (H9). (B) Embryoid bodies (EB) at day 9 of differentiation. (C) Neuroepithelium appear at day 12. (D) Neuroepithelium appear as translucent bright rings at day 12. (E) Optic vesicle/cup at day 21. (F) Neural retinal (NR) region at day 26. Scale bars: 1000 µm (A, D, and E); 400 µm (B and C); 200 µm (F). All photos are provided by Dr. Ze-Hua Xu.

they develop into optic vesicles (**Figure 2E**), followed by neuroretinas (**Figure 2F**), which in turn differentiate into seven types of retinal cells. The sequence of retinal cell types is consistent with in vivo development [36]. After differentiation, the cells undergo spontaneous nuclear migration, forming pinnacles and finally arranged into layered structures, in which the ganglion cells are located in the inner layer of the retinal organoid and the photoreceptors are located in the outer layer of the retinal organoid [26, 27]. Since RPE is usually a mass of cells not adjacent to the neuroretina and is not derived from the floating culture of optic vesicles, we do not consider it to be part of the retinoid organoid in this paper. With the continuous development of differentiation technology, photoreceptors in organoids become more and more mature, which is manifested by the appearance of outer segments and photosensitivity [37, 38].

3. Differentiation of retinal organoids

The development of retinal organoid technology is the result of continuous attempts and innovations by a large number of researchers. Here, we try to review the progress of retinal organoids differentiation in the past ten years (**Figure 3**).

3.1 Diversity of differentiation methods

There are various differentiation methods for retinal organoids, but in terms of differentiation steps, there are mainly two differentiation schemes (**Figure 4**). The first is a classic 3D differentiation protocol from Sassi's team [26, 27]. The stem cells were dissociated and reassembled in a serum-free and low-growth factor medium (SFEBq culture, or serum-free culture of embryoid body-like aggregates with quick aggregation), and forced to form an embryoid body (EB) in a 96-well V-shaped plate.

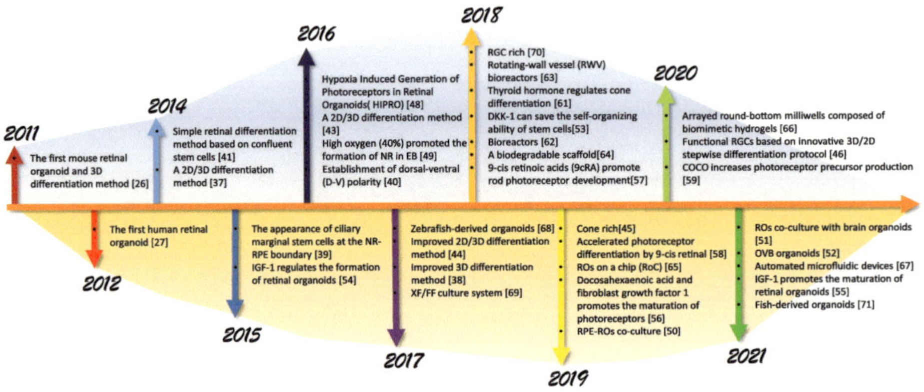

Figure 3.
Progress in retinal organoid differentiation over the decade.

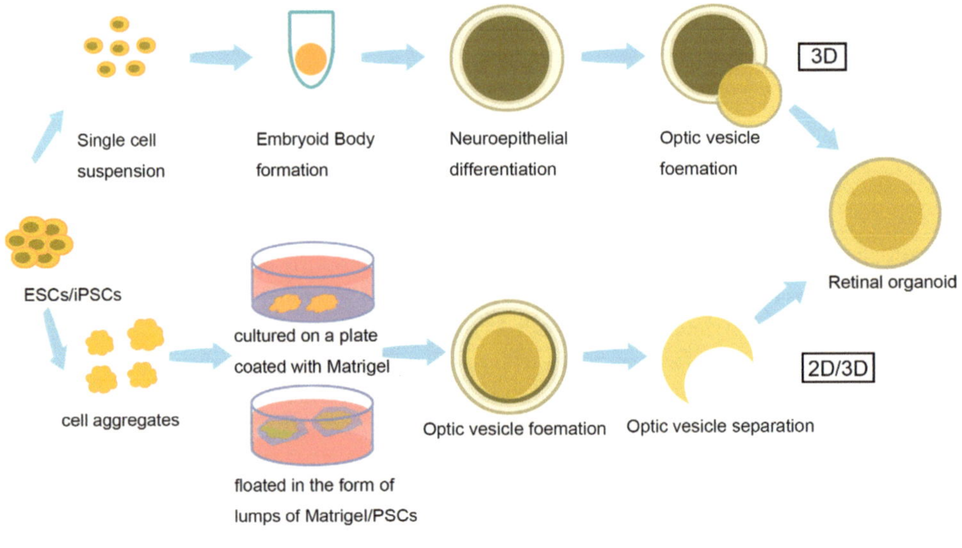

Figure 4.
Two main methods of retinal organoid differentiation.

They were then stimulated by the addition of Matrigel to differentiate into neuroepithelial cells and subsequently into retinal progenitor cells and double-layer optic cup structures [27]. The cells were in suspension culture during the whole process of differentiation, and the formation of optic cups and the differentiation of neuroretina were self-organized [27]. 3D differentiation protocol is complicated in the early stage of differentiation, but it has a higher degree of reduction in the retinal development process, including the occurrence of optic cups invagination, the appearance of ciliary marginal stem cells at the NR-RPE boundary [39], and the establishment of dorsal-ventral (D-V) polarity [40].

The second differentiation method combines 2D culture and 3D culture (2D/3D) [37, 41–46], and the difference is mainly reflected in the early stage of neural induction. It has been reported that pluripotent stem cells can differentiate into the retina even when they are simply fused together [41, 42]. In this differentiation scheme, the stem cells were divided into small pieces by enzymatic hydrolysis [37] or mechanical methods [41, 43, 45] to form aggregates. The aggregates were cultured on a plate coated with Matrigel or floated in medium in the form of lumps of Matrigel/PSCs [43, 45]. After it differentiated into neuroepithelium and optic vesicles, the latter were separated for suspension culture and further differentiated into retinal organoids. This approach bypasses EB formation stage and induces optic vesicle formation by endogenous production of inducer molecules from aggregated cells, avoiding the aggregation step of SFEBq method and the need of Wnt/BMP antagonist [47]. These studies suggest that cell-cell and cell-extracellular matrix interactions are key to inducing retinal organoids differentiation in the early stage of stem cell differentiation.

With the improvement of differentiation methods, the structure of retinal organoids has been improved. Photoreceptors can reach advanced maturity, characterized by the formation of the inner and outer segments and connecting cilia of photoreceptors, the appearance of photosensitivity [37, 44], the expression of photoreceptor neurotransmitters, and the formation of synaptic bands [38, 44]. By adjusting the differentiation method, we can also change the proportion of cells in organoids, such as retinal organoids rich in cones or RGCs [45, 46], which is good for cell transplantation. Oxygen is also an important factor in regulating the differentiation of retinal organoids, and hypoxic conditions (5%) effectively produce vesicles and cups as well as more mature neuroretinas [48]. Another study showed that high oxygen (40%) promoted the formation of NR in EB, as well as the generation, migration and maturation of retinal ganglion cells during metaphase differentiation [49]. The co-culture of RPE with retinal organoids promoted the differentiation of photoreceptors [50], while the co-culture with brain organoids promoted the axon extension of RGCs [51]. More encouragingly, researchers have differentiated human brain organoids with bilaterally symmetric vesicles [52].

3.2 Modulation of signaling molecules

Retinal development requires the regulation of a series of signaling molecules. Similarly, by adding different signaling molecules, retinal organoids differentiation can be regulated in vitro. Dickkopf-related protein 1 (DKK-1), a Wnt signaling pathway antagonist, salvages the self-organizing ability of stem cells to differentiate into retinal progenitor cells [53]. Insulin-like growth factor 1 (IGF-1) regulates the formation of retinal organoids and promotes the formation of the correct retinal lamellar structure by various retinal cells [54, 55]. In the absence of IGF-1, retinal lamination was absent at the early stage of differentiation, while photoreceptors decreased and retinal ganglion cells increased at the late stage of differentiation [55]. Addition of docosahexaenoic acid and fibroblast growth factor 1 can specifically promote the maturation of photoreceptors including cones [56]. Replacement of widely used all-trans retinoic acid with 9-cis-retinoic acid in culture medium promoted the expression of rod photoreceptors rhodopsin and the maturation of mitochondrial morphology [57, 58]. COCO protein can block BMP/TGFβ/Wnt signaling pathway, enhance photoreceptor precursors, and promote s-cone differentiation and inner segment protuberances formation [59, 60]. During retinal development, s-cone appear first, followed by L/M-cones. This time transition from the designation of the s-cone to the production of the L/M-cone is controlled by thyroid hormone (TH) signaling [61].

3.3 Combination of organoid technology and tissue engineering technology

There is also a lot of innovative research that combines retinal organoid technology with emerging materials technology. The use of bioreactors improved retinal stratification and increased the production of photoreceptors with cilia and new outer segments [62]. In static culture, the development of retinal organoids may be limited by oxygen and nutrient diffusion, and rotating-wall vessel (RWV) bioreactors can accelerate and improve the growth and differentiation of retinal organoids [63]. The spherical structure of retinal organoids limits its interaction with host RPE and the remaining neuroretinas during transplantation. In order to create a planar retinal organoid, a biodegradable scaffold was developed that mimics the extracellular matrix of neuroretinas [64]. Retina-on-a-chip is a new microphysiological model of the human retina that integrates seven different basic retinal cell types and provides vascular-like perfusion to retinal organoids [65]. Arrayed bottom-lined micropores composed of bionic hydrogels, facilitated rapid retinoid tissue formation from mESCs aggregates in an efficient and routine manner [66]. Automated microfluidic devices with significantly reduced shear stress can maintain the long-term survival of retinal organoids [67]. For details of some other differentiation improvements [68–71], please refer to **Figure 3**.

4. Applications of retinal organoids

As a three-dimensional multicellular structure formed by self-organization in vitro, retinal organoids can reproduce the development process of retina in vivo to some extent, and can be used to summarize some structural and functional characteristics of human retina. Meanwhile, they are the most promising tools for retinal disease research (**Figure 5**).

4.1 Retinal organoids as disease models

The reprogramming technique enables iPSCs-derived retinal organoids to retain the patient's genetic characteristics, allowing us to study a variety of retinal diseases in detail in a dish. To date, retinitis pigmentosa (RP), Laber congenital amaurosis (LCA), retinoblastoma (RB) and some other retinal diseases (**Table 1**) have been reproduced in dishes using retinal organoid technology [47, 98].

RP is a relatively common hereditary retinal disorder characterized by night blindness and progressive loss of visual field [99]. LCA, the main disease leading to

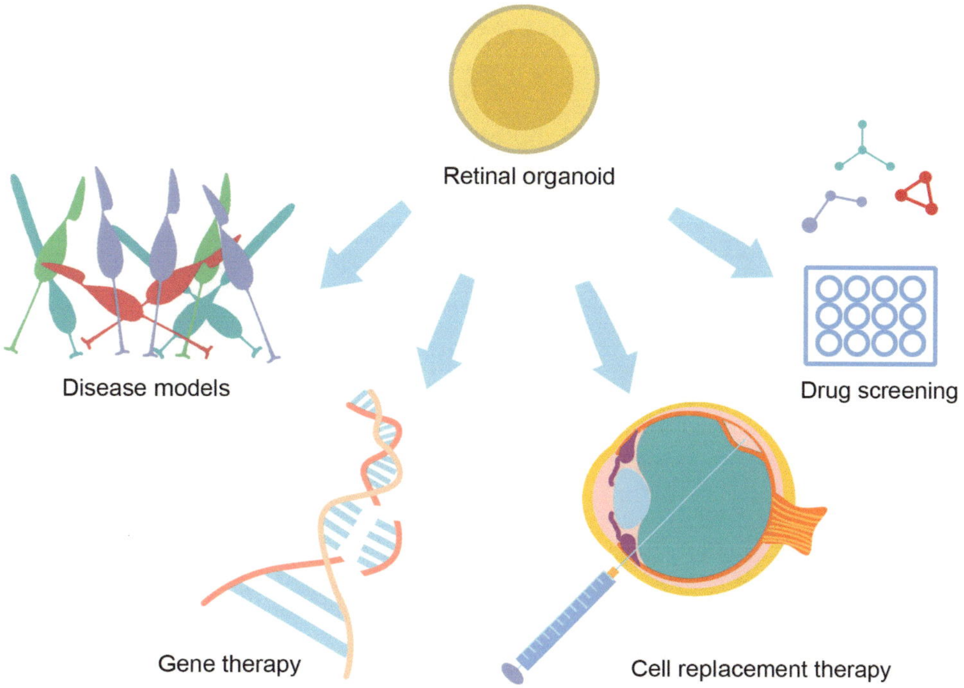

Figure 5.
Applications of retinal organoids.

Disease models	Genetic mutations	Phenotypes of retinal organoids	Reference
RP	Rp11(PRPF31 gene mutation)	Gradually degenerating photoreceptors; disrupted cilia morphology	[72]
RP	RPGR gene frameshift mutation	Photoreceptors have significant defects in morphology, localization, transcription profile and electrophysiological activity; shorted cilium was found in patient retinal organoids	[73]
RP	RP17 structural variants	Increased GDPD1 expression may lead to dysregulation of lipid metabolism, thus affecting photoreceptor function	[74]
RP	USH2A gene mutation	Aberrant organoids polarization, defective neuroepithelium, and abnormal RPCs and photoceptors differentiation	[75]
RP	Crb1 gene mutation	Small but frequent disruptions of CRB complex members at the outer limiting membrane	[76]
RP	PDE6B gene mutation	Increased cGMP levels	[77]
RP	TRNT1 gene mutation	Reduced levels of full-length TRNT1 protein and expression of a truncated smaller protein; autophagy was defective, with abnormal accumulation of LC3-II and elevated oxidative stress levels	[78]

Disease models	Genetic mutations	Phenotypes of retinal organoids	Reference
RP	USH2A gene mutation	Post-developmental photoreceptor degeneration	[79]
RP	REEP6 gene mutation	The expression of a retina-specific isoform REEP6.1 changes destabilize the protein	[80]
XLRP	RP2 gene mutation	Rod cell death peaked at day 150 and the outer nuclear layer thinned at day 180	[81]
LCA	CRX gene mutation	Defective photoreceptor maturation with diminished expression of visual opsins	[82]
LCA	RPE65 gene mutation	Lower expression of RPE65, but similar phagocytic activity and VEGF secretion level	[83]
LCA	AIPL1 gene mutation	Patient-derived organoids maintained retinal cell cytoarchitecture despite significantly reduced levels of AIPL1	[84]
LCA	CEP290 gene mutation	Cilia defects were evident in photoreceptors	[85]
LCA	CEP290 gene mutation	A high level of aberrant splicing and cilia defects	[86]
LCA	CRX gene mutation	Immature and dysfunctional photoreceptor cells	[87]
LCA	CEP290 gene mutation	CEP290 aberrant splicing	[88]
RB	RB1 double allele deletion	Homozygous deletion of RB1 did not affect the maturation and proliferation statuses of human iPSCs (no ROs phenotype)	[89]
RB	RB1 double allele mutation or deletion	Rb originated from ARR3-positive maturing cone precursors during development; tumorigenesis in retinal organoids	[90]
RB	RB1 germline mutation	Retinoblastomas formed from retinal organoids have molecular, cellular and genomic features indistinguishable from human retinoblastomas	[91]
S-cone syndrome	NRL loss	Two distinct populations of s-opsin expressing photoreceptors emerge; one population more representative of typical cones, and the other of rod/cone intermediates	[92]
Rod-cone dystrophy	CRB1 gene mutation	A novel CRB1 transcript displaying skipping of exon 6	[93]
Macular telangiectasia type 2	Normal organoids were treated with deoxy	Dead photoreceptors	[94]
Microphthalmia	VSX2(R200Q) gene mutation	Bipolar cells are absent; delayed photoreceptor maturation	[95]
Stargardt disease	ABCA4 gene mutation	ABCA4 splicing defect	[96]
X-linked juvenile cleft retina (XLRS)	RS1 gene mutation	Retinal splitting, defective retinoschisin production, outer-segment defects, abnormal paxillin turnover, and impaired ER-Golgi transportation	[97]

Table 1.
Retinal organoids as disease models.

congenital blindness in infants, accounts for more than 5% of hereditary retinopathy, with complete loss of binocular cone and rod function within 1 year after birth [100]. Both diseases have been reported to be associated with multiple pathogenic genes. By differentiating different genetically-mutated stem cell lines into retinal organoids [101], we can observe their disease phenotypes in dishes, including photoreceptor degeneration, ciliary morphology disorder, and various functional impairment at molecular levels. Retinoblastoma is the most common intraocular malignancy in children [102]. The main cause of retinoblastoma is the loss of RB1 gene expression [103]. RB1 gene is a tumor suppressor gene, but the mechanism of RB1 deletion leading to retinal cancer is not clear, one of the key questions is the origin of RB cancer. By constructing RB models based on retinal organoids [104], we successfully observed tumorigenesis in retinal organoids and demonstrated that RB originates from ARR3 positive precursors of mature cones during development [90]. Other disease models, such as s-cone syndrome, rod-cone dystrophy, Macular telangiectasia type 2, microphthalmia, Stargardt disease, X-linked juvenile cleft retina, have also contributed to our understanding of retinal diseases.

4.2 Retinal organoids as tools for therapeutic research

4.2.1 Gene therapy

Identification of pathogenic genes promotes the generation of animal models and elucidates the physiological functions of gene products to a certain extent, thus promoting the development of gene therapy. So far, most research has focused on saving retinal organoid disease phenotypes through gene editing of patient-specific induced pluripotent stem cells [72, 73, 87, 97, 105, 106]. However, this strategy cannot be applied to patients. Adeno-associated virus (AAV) show great promise as a gene therapy vector for a wide range of retinal diseases. For example, AAV-mediated gene augmentation has successfully treated LCA caused by RPE65 mutations [107]. AAV-mediated gene therapy based on retinal organoids has also shown promising results in the laboratory [81, 82, 108]. In addition, gene therapies such as antisense morpholino and antisense oligonucleotides (AONs) have also been reported (**Table 2**).

4.2.2 Cell replacement therapy

Hereditary retinal degenerative diseases such as RP, Stargardt's disease and LCA are the leading cause of incurable blindness. The vision loss associated with these diseases is caused by the death of photoreceptors in the retina. Existing treatments, including neuroprotection and gene therapy, require the presence of endogenous photoreceptors. In addition, due to the complex mechanism of retinal degeneration diseases, especially RP, it has been found that there are multiple genes with multiple mutation modes, and treatment methods focusing on a single mutation are extremely difficult technically and economically. Thus, transplant-based photoreceptor cell replacement becomes an attractive therapeutic strategy for restoring visual function and, if successful, could be applied to a wide range of retinal degenerative diseases.

Research on retinal cell transplantation dates back to 2006 [109]. Mice were able to effectively integrate rod photoreceptor precursor cells isolated from juvenile mice retinas into the ONL. These cells can further differentiate in the host retina and exhibit morphological characteristics typical of mature photoreceptors, such as inner and outer segments, while expressing molecules necessary for light transduction,

ROs	Gene therapy	Result	Reference
CEP290-LCA-Optic Cups	Antisense morpholino	Effectively blocked aberrant splicing and restored expression of full-length CEP290, restoring normal cilia-based protein trafficking	[86]
RP11 (PRPF31)-RP-ROs	CRISPR/Cas9-mediated gene correction	Rescued protein expression and key cellular phenotypes in RPE and photoreceptors	[72]
RPGR-RP-ROs	CRISPR/Cas9-mediated gene correction	Rescued photoreceptor structure and electrophysiological property, reversed the observed ciliopathy	[73]
CEP290-LCA10-ROs	Antisense oligonucleotides	Restored wild-type CEP290 mRNA and protein expression levels	[88]
CEP290-Rd16-mROs	AAV-mediated CEP290 fragment	Improved cilia phenotype	[108]
RS1-XLRS-ROs	CRISPR/Cas9-mediated base-editing	Normalized the splitting phenotype, outer-segment defects, paxillin dynamics, ciliary marker expression, and transcriptome profiles	[97]
RP2KO-XLRP-ROs	AAV-mediated gene augmentation	Rescued the degeneration phenotype of the RP2 KO organoids, to prevent ONL thinning and restore rhodopsin expression	[81]
ABCA4-Stargardt-ROs	Antisense oligonucleotides(AONs)	Saved the splicing defect	[96]
G56R-ADRP-ROs	CRISPR/Cas9 mediated gene knockout	ROs differentiation and NR2E3 expression were normal	[106]
CRX-LCA-ROs	AAV-mediated CRX gene augmentation therapy	Partially restored photoreceptor phenotype and expression of phototransduction-related genes; Reduced the loss of opsin expression	[82]
CLN3-RP-ROs	Gene correction	Restored CLN3 mRNA and protein expression and prevented SCMAS and inner segment vacuolization	[105]
CRX-LCA7-ROs	CRISPR/Cas9-based gene knockout	Rescued the photoreceptor phenotypes in organoids	[87]

Table 2.
Gene therapy based on retinal organoids.

forming synaptic connections with downstream cells, generating light responses and promoting visual function [109–115]. These results demonstrate the feasibility of photoreceptor transplantation as a therapeutic strategy for restoring visual acuity after retinal degeneration.

However, this cannot be applied to the treatment of retinal diseases in humans. There are ethical challenges to primary photoreceptors transplantation, but stem cell-based photoreceptors can avoid this problem. It has been shown that photoreceptor cells derived from stem cells can be integrated into mouse retinas, restoring the animal's response to light [116, 117]. This is far from enough, until the appearance of retinal organoids, retinal cell transplantation and clinical transformation have made a breakthrough.

Transplantation of retinal organoids, mainly photoreceptors, is also a process of constant exploration [118]. The safety and effectiveness of transplantation, the enrichment and purification of transplanted cells, the effects of retinal organoids at different stages of development and host retinas with different degrees of degeneration on the efficiency of transplantation, and the evaluation of cell integration and function after transplantation are all issues that need to be explored.

Table 3 gives a brief summary of some retinal organoid transplantation cases in recent years. There are two transplantation methods: one is to digest the retinal

Graft/Host	Transplantation method	Transplantation result	Reference
Rhodopsin-GFP-mESC-ROs-rod precursors/adult mice with retinal degeneration	Cell suspension	Transplanted cells integrate within the degenerated retinas of mice and mature into outer segment-bearing photoreceptors	[119]
CRX-GFP-mESC-ROs-photoreceptors/adult NOD/SCID recipient mice	Cell suspension	After transplantation, the integrated cells showed typical mature rod structures with outer segments and banded synapses	[120]
mESC or miPSC-derived 3D retinal tissue/advanced retinal degeneration model (rd1) that lacked ONL	Retinal tissue	A structured outer nuclear layer (ONL) with complete inner and outer segments was developed; host-graft synaptic connections were observed	[121]
hESC-retina sheet/ Two focal selective photoreceptor degeneration monkey models	Retinal tissue	Transplanted retinal tissue differentiated into a series of retinal cell types, including rod and cone photoreceptors that formed structured outer nuclear layers; formation of host-graft synaptic connections	[122]
Rhodopsin-GFP-mESC-ROs-(CD73-MACS)-photoreceptors/mouse models with mild or severe cone-rod degeneration	Cell suspension	Some cells integrated into mouse retinas and acquired a mature morphology, expressing rod and synaptic markers in close proximity to secondary neurons	[123]
Mesc-ROs-cone/adult Aipl1−/− mice	Cell suspension	Transplanted cells showed capacity to survive and mature in the subretinal space	[124]
hPSC-ROs-L/M-opsin+ cones/Nrl−/−mice or advanced retinal degeneration mice	Cell suspension	Human cones can become incorporated within an adult mammalian retina	[44]
hiPSC-ROs(cGMP)-photoreceptors/ immunodeficient mouse	Cell suspension	Retinal cells successfully integrated into the photoreceptor layer and developed into mature photoreceptors	[125]
hESC-ROs-retinal sheets/ mice of end-stage retinal degeneration with immunodeficiency	Retinal tissue	Long-term survival and well-structured graft photoreceptor layer maturation without rejection or tumor formation; formation of host-graft synaptic connections	[126]
hESC-ROs(30–65 days of differentiation)-retinal sheets/immunodeficient rho S334ter-3 rats	Retinal tissue	The transplanted sheets differentiated, integrated, and produced functional photoreceptors and other retinal cells; maturation of the transplanted retinal cells created visual improvements; the donor cells were synaptically active	[127]

Graft/Host	Transplantation method	Transplantation result	Reference
CRX-hiPSC-ROs-photoreceptors precursors (CD73-MACS)/P23H rats	Cell suspension	CD73+ photoreceptor precursors can be isolated in large numbers and transplanted into rat eyes, showing capacity to survive and mature in close proximity to host inner retina (hiPSC-derived retinal cells did not appear to migrate to host ONL)	[128]
CRX-hiPSC-ROs-photoreceptors precursors/Pde6brd1 mice	Cell suspension	The CRX+ cells settled next to the inner nuclear layer and made connections with the inner neurons of the host retina, and approximately one-third of them expressed the pan cone marker, Arrestin 3, indicating further maturation upon integration into the host retina	[129]
hESC-ROs-retinal progenitor cells (RPCs)/RD models of rats and mice	Cell suspension	Transplanted cells significantly improve vision and preserve the retinal structure	[130]
hiPSC-ROs-Jaws-expressing PRs/blind mice lacking the photoreceptor layer	Cell suspension	Light-driven responses at the photoreceptor and ganglion cell levels were observed	[131]
hiPSCs-ROs-Müller glia/rats depleted of retinal ganglion cells by NMDA	Cell suspension	Transplanted cells can partially restore visual function	[132]
hESC-ROs-retinal tissue/cat	Retinal tissue	Large number of graft-derived fibers connecting the graft and the host; presence of human-specific synaptophysin puncta in the cat retina	[133]
hESC-Ros-retinal sheet/immunodeficient RCS rats	Retinal tissue	The transplanted organoids survived more than 7 months; developed photoreceptors with inner and outer segments, and other retinal cells; and were well-integrated within the host	[134]
hiPSC-ROs-cones/mice with retinal degeneration	Cell suspension	Restoration of surprisingly complex light-evoked retinal ganglion cell responses and improved light-evoked behaviors in treated animals	[135]
hiPSC-ROs-retinal sheets with PLGA scaffolds/rhesus monkey	Retinal tissue	With sufficient graft-host contact provided by the scaffold, the transplanted tissues survived for up to 1 year without tumorigenesis; Histological examinations indicated survival, further maturation, and migration	[136]
mESC-ROs-retinal progenitor cells (RPC)/mice with retinal degeneration	Cell suspension	RPC grafts form active synaptic networks within sites of ADR that functionally integrate with the retinal neuron populations and that resemble physiological patterns of neural circuits to the normal retina	[137]

Graft/Host	Transplantation method	Transplantation result	Reference
ROs and polarized RPE sheets were made into a co-graft using bio-adhesives/ immunodeficient RCS rats	Total retina patch	Co-grafts grew, generated new photoreceptors and developed neuronal processes that were integrated into the host retina	[138]

Table 3.
Research on transplantation of retinal organoids.

organ into a single cell, from which the photoreceptor cells are purified and enriched, and the transplantation is carried out in the form of cell suspension. Another method is to strip the photoreceptor layer from the retinal organ and transplant it in thin slices. This method is more difficult to operate, because it is difficult to maintain the correct shape and polarity of the retina when it is transplanted into the eye of the host, and appropriate transplantation instruments need to be designed. The implant may contain some interneurons that block the connection between photoreceptor cells and the remaining inner layer of the retina in the host, and there are eye size requirements in the host animal. The implant is usually performed in rats, cats and non-human primates. In general, we have gained a lot from the exploration of retinal organ transplantation. A number of studies have shown that transplanted cells or tissues can survive in the host eye for a long time, migrate and integrate into the correct location. Integrated cells can further differentiate and mature in vivo, presenting typical cell structures, such as internal and external segments, and expressing corresponding cell markers and synaptic markers. In some studies, the formation of synaptic connections between host and graft and improvement of host visual function were also observed. In the host, transplanted cells or tissues are electrically excitatory [136], indicating their potential for restoring visual function. Through behavioral and electrophysiological experiments, we found that the host can not only slow down the progressive visual loss to some extent, but also show a relatively significant recovery of visual function [127, 130, 131, 134, 135, 137, 138]. These are exciting results and suggest that cell replacement therapy based on retinal organoids is a promising treatment that will bring light to patients with retinal diseases.

4.3 Retinal organoids for drug screening

Drug development focuses on screening, a process that requires cell models. The closer the cell model was to the physiological state, the more accurate the screening was. Therefore, organoids are undoubtedly a better choice for drug screening. Some ocular supplements, vitamin E, lutein, astaxanthin, and anthocyanin, have been reported to protect retinal photoreceptor degeneration induced by 4-hydroxytamoxifen (4-OHT) and light [139]. Few studies have successfully screened effective drugs using retinal organoids. In addition, there are some studies using retinal organoids as screening tools to explore the membrane transport effects of some microbial opsin [140]. These results suggest that retinal organoids can be used to validate the effectiveness of some therapeutic products and drug molecules.

5. Limitations and deficiencies

In recent years, although the technology of retinal organoids has made great progress, it is still beyond the reach of our existing tools and technologies to construct retinal organoids with the same structure and physiological functions as the mature retina in vivo. Our research on retinal organoids is still in its infancy and there are some limitations to overcome.

Long-term maintenance of retinal organoids depends on oxygen and nutrients, and in our existing culture system, oxygen diffusion limits the size of retinal organoids and the development of their internal cells, especially ganglion cells. Currently, we are trying to introduce a combination of tissue engineering techniques to solve this problem, such as the use of bioreactors and retinal chips [62, 63, 65]. The absence of vascular system also limits the long-term maintenance of organoids. Microglia are the resident immune cells of the central nervous system and are particularly important for the development of the retina, which can regulate the survival of neurons and prune synapses [141]. Co-differentiation of retinal organoids and vascular tissues or microglia in a dish is challenging because they come from different germ layers. The retina develops from the ectoderm, while vascular tissue-associated cells and microglia originate from the mesoderm. Therefore, we usually choose to achieve the complexity of retinal organoids through co-culture. In recent years, the realization of vascular structure in human brain has made some progress. After transplantation of human cerebral organs into the cerebral cortex of mice, the growth of blood vessels in mice was induced to increase the survival and maturation of cells [142]. In vitro, a study found that ectopic expression of human ETS variant 2 (ETV2) in hESCs can form a complex vascular-like network in human cortical organs and promote the maturation of organoid function [143]. In the future, we also expect that 3D printing of vascular tissue [144] and co-culture with mesodermal progenitor cells [145] will make the differentiation system of retinal organoids more perfect. For the retina in a petri dish to function, the most important point is to establish synaptic connections and form functional circuits. While our differentiated retina can form synaptic connections now, it's not nearly as good as the complex network of synapses in the retina in vivo. Even retinal organoids derived from normal stem cell lines respond poorly to light. This may be due to the gradual degeneration of ganglion cells during late differentiation and lack of connection to the brain, which hindrance our assessment of retinal functional circuits. It may also be associated with limited growth of the outer segment due to the lack of direct interaction with RPE. Retinal organoid technology has solved the problem of cell-cell interaction, but in organisms, tissue-to-tissue and organ-to-organ interactions remain important for development. For example, the relationship of the retina to the lens, ciliary body and cornea, and the relationship of the retina to the brain.

6. Conclusions

It's an exciting time, and technological advances have made a lot of things possible. Retinal organoids are our research tools for overcoming retinal diseases. It allows us to further understand the development and maturation of the retina, reproduce disease pathology and phenotypes in vitro, and explore the feasibility of gene therapy. In addition, it provides us with cells for cell transplantation and drug screening. We have enjoyed the great benefits brought by retinal organoids. However, their defects and deficiencies are also prominent, which is the direction we need to work towards. There is still a long way to go in the development of retinal organoids, and we expect that technological breakthroughs will enable us to advance to the next level in this field in the future.

Acknowledgements

We thank Dr. Ze-Hua Xu for providing photos of retinal organoid differentiation.

Author details

Jing Yuan and Zi-Bing Jin*
Beijing Institute of Ophthalmology, Beijing Tongren Eye Center, Beijing Tongren Hospital, Capital Medical University, Beijing Ophthalmology and Visual Science Key Laboratory, Beijing, China

*Address all correspondence to: jinzibing@foxmail.com

References

[1] Demb JB, Singer JH. Functional circuitry of the retina. Annual Review of Vision Science. 2015;**1**:263-289. DOI: 10.1146/annurev-vision-082114-035334

[2] Reese BE. Development of the retina and optic pathway. Vision Research. 2011;**51**:613-632. DOI: 10.1016/j.visres.2010.07.010

[3] Masland RH. The neuronal organization of the retina. Neuron. 2012;**76**:266-280. DOI: 10.1016/j.neuron.2012.10.002

[4] Bumsted O'Brien KM, Cheng H, Jiang Y, Schulte D, Swaroop A, Hendrickson AE. Expression of photoreceptor-specific nuclear receptor NR2E3 in rod photoreceptors of fetal human retina. Investigative Ophthalmology & Visual Science. 2004;**45**:2807-2812. DOI: 10.1167/iovs.03-1317

[5] McLeod DS, Hasegawa T, Prow T, Merges C, Lutty G. The initial fetal human retinal vasculature develops by vasculogenesis. Developmental Dynamics. 2006;**235**:3336-3347. DOI: 10.1002/dvdy.20988

[6] Bell CM, Zack DJ, Berlinicke CA. Human organoids for the study of retinal development and disease. Annual Review of Vision Science. 2020;**6**:91-114. DOI: 10.1146/annurev-vision-121219-081855

[7] Szatko KP, Korympidou MM, Ran Y, Berens P, Dalkara D, Schubert T, et al. Neural circuits in the mouse retina support color vision in the upper visual field. Nature Communications. 2020;**11**:3481. DOI: 10.1038/s41467-020-17113-8

[8] Masuda T, Zhang X, Berlinicke C, Wan J, Yerrabelli A, Conner EA, et al. The transcription factor GTF2IRD1 regulates the topology and function of photoreceptors by modulating photoreceptor gene expression across the retina. The Journal of Neuroscience. 2014;**34**:15356-15368. DOI: 10.1523/JNEUROSCI.2089-14.2014

[9] Ortin-Martinez A, Nadal-Nicolas FM, Jimenez-Lopez M, Alburquerque-Bejar JJ, Nieto-Lopez L, Garcia-Ayuso D, et al. Number and distribution of mouse retinal cone photoreceptors: Differences between an albino (Swiss) and a pigmented (C57/BL6) strain. PLoS One. 2014;**9**:e102392. DOI: 10.1371/journal.pone.0102392

[10] Volland S, Esteve-Rudd J, Hoo J, Yee C, Williams DS. A comparison of some organizational characteristics of the mouse central retina and the human macula. PLoS One. 2015;**10**:e0125631. DOI: 10.1371/journal.pone.0125631

[11] Peng YR, Shekhar K, Yan W, Herrmann D, Sappington A, Bryman GS, et al. Molecular classification and comparative Taxonomics of foveal and peripheral cells in primate retina. Cell. 2019;**176**(1222-1237):e1222. DOI: 10.1016/j.cell.2019.01.004

[12] Provis JM, Dubis AM, Maddess T, Carroll J. Adaptation of the central retina for high acuity vision: Cones, the fovea and the avascular zone. Progress in Retinal and Eye Research. 2013;**35**:63-81. DOI: 10.1016/j.preteyeres.2013.01.005

[13] Thomson JA, Itskovitz-Eldor J, Shapiro SS, Waknitz MA, Swiergiel JJ, Marshall VS, et al. Embryonic stem cell lines derived from human blastocysts. Science. 1998;**282**:1145-1147. DOI: 10.1126/science.282.5391.1145

[14] Takahashi K, Tanabe K, Ohnuki M, Narita M, Ichisaka T, Tomoda K, et al. Induction of pluripotent stem cells from adult human fibroblasts by defined factors. Cell. 2007;**131**:861-872. DOI: 10.1016/j.cell.2007.11.019

[15] Banin E, Obolensky A, Idelson M, Hemo I, Reinhardtz E, Pikarsky E, et al. Retinal incorporation and differentiation of neural precursors derived from human embryonic stem cells. Stem Cells. 2006;**24**:246-257. DOI: 10.1634/stemcells.2005-0009

[16] Lamba DA, Karl MO, Ware CB, Reh TA. Efficient generation of retinal progenitor cells from human embryonic stem cells. Proceedings of the National Academy of Sciences. 2006;**103**:12769-12774

[17] Mukhopadhyay M, Shtrom S, Rodriguez-Esteban C, Chen L, Tsukui T, Gomer L, et al. Dickkopf1 is required for embryonic head induction and limb morphogenesis in the mouse. Developmental Cell. 2001;**1**:423-434

[18] Zhou S, Flamier A, Abdouh M, Tetreault N, Barabino A, Wadhwa S, et al. Differentiation of human embryonic stem cells into cone photoreceptors through simultaneous inhibition of BMP. TGFbeta and Wnt Signaling. Development. 2015;**142**: 3294-3306. DOI: 10.1242/dev.125385

[19] Uygun BE, Sharma N, Yarmush M. Retinal pigment epithelium differentiation of stem cells: Current status and challenges. Critical Reviews in Biomedical Engineering. 2009;**37**:355-375. DOI: 10.1615/critrevbiomedeng.v37.i4-5.30

[20] Sluch VM, Chamling X, Liu MM, Berlinicke CA, Cheng J, Mitchell KL, et al. Enhanced stem cell differentiation and Immunopurification of genome engineered human retinal ganglion cells. Stem Cells Translational Medicine. 2017;**6**:1972-1986. DOI: 10.1002/sctm.17-0059

[21] Osakada F, Ikeda H, Mandai M, Wataya T, Watanabe K, Yoshimura N, et al. Toward the generation of rod and cone photoreceptors from mouse, monkey and human embryonic stem cells. Nature Biotechnology. 2008;**26**: 215-224. DOI: 10.1038/nbt1384

[22] Keller G. Embryonic stem cell differentiation: Emergence of a new era in biology and medicine. Genes & Development. 2005;**19**:1129-1155. DOI: 10.1101/gad.1303605

[23] Jin Z-B, Takahashi M. Generation of retinal cells from pluripotent stem cells. Progress in Brain Research. 2012;**201**:171-181

[24] Jin Z-B, Okamoto S, Mandai M, Takahashi M. Induced pluripotent stem cells for retinal degenerative diseases: A new perspective on the challenges. Journal of Genetics. 2009;**88**:417-424

[25] Jin Z-B, Okamoto S, Osakada F, Homma K, Assawachananont J, Hirami Y, et al. Modeling retinal degeneration using patient-specific induced pluripotent stem cells. PloS One. 2011;**6**:e17084

[26] Eiraku M, Takata N, Ishibashi H, Kawada M, Sakakura E, Okuda S, et al. Self-organizing optic-cup morphogenesis in three-dimensional culture. Nature. 2011;**472**:51-56. DOI: 10.1038/nature09941

[27] Nakano T, Ando S, Takata N, Kawada M, Muguruma K, Sekiguchi K, et al. Self-formation of optic cups and storable stratified neural retina from human ESCs. Cell Stem Cell. 2012;**10**:771-785. DOI: 10.1016/j.stem.2012.05.009

[28] Zuber ME, Gestri G, Viczian AS, Barsacchi G, Harris WA. Specification of the vertebrate eye by a network of eye field transcription factors. Development. 2003;**130**:5155-5167. DOI: 10.1242/dev.00723

[29] O'Rahilly R, Muller F. Developmental stages in human embryos: Revised and new measurements. Cells, Tissues, Organs. 2010;**192**:73-84. DOI: 10.1159/000289817

[30] Müller F, O'Rahilly RJA. The first appearance of the neural tube and optic primordium in the human embryo at stage. Anatomy and Embryology. 1985;**172**:157-169

[31] Pearson AA. The development of the eyelids. Part I. External features. Journal of Anatomy. 1980;**130**:33

[32] Perron M, Kanekar S, Vetter ML, Harris WA. The genetic sequence of retinal development in the ciliary margin of theXenopusEye. Developmental Biology. 1998;**199**:185-200

[33] Cepko CL, Austin CP, Yang X, Alexiades M, Ezzeddine D. Cell fate determination in the vertebrate retina. Proceedings of the National Academy of Sciences. 1996;**93**:589-595

[34] Blanks JC, Adinolfi AM, Lolley RN. Synaptogenesis in the photoreceptor terminal of the mouse retina. Journal of Comparative Neurology. 1974;**156**:81-93

[35] Fisher LJ. Development of synaptic arrays in the inner plexiform layer of neonatal mouse retina. Journal of Comparative Neurology. 1979;**187**:359-372

[36] O'Hara-Wright M, Gonzalez-Cordero A. Retinal organoids: A window into human retinal development. Development. 2020;**147**. DOI: 10.1242/dev.189746

[37] Zhong X, Gutierrez C, Xue T, Hampton C, Vergara MN, Cao LH, et al. Generation of three-dimensional retinal tissue with functional photoreceptors from human iPSCs. Nature Communications. 2014;**5**:4047. DOI: 10.1038/ncomms5047

[38] Wahlin KJ, Maruotti JA, Sripathi SR, Ball J, Angueyra JM, Kim C, et al. Photoreceptor outer segment-like structures in long-term 3D retinas from human pluripotent stem cells. Scientific Reports. 2017;**7**:766. DOI: 10.1038/s41598-017-00774-9

[39] Kuwahara A, Ozone C, Nakano T, Saito K, Eiraku M, Sasai Y. Generation of a ciliary margin-like stem cell niche from self-organizing human retinal tissue. Nature Communications. 2015;**6**:6286. DOI: 10.1038/ncomms7286

[40] Hasegawa Y, Takata N, Okuda S, Kawada M, Eiraku M, Sasai Y. Emergence of dorsal-ventral polarity in ES cell-derived retinal tissue. Development. 2016;**143**: 3895-3906. DOI: 10.1242/dev.134601

[41] Reichman S, Terray A, Slembrouck A, Nanteau C, Orieux G, Habeler W, et al. From confluent human iPS cells to self-forming neural retina and retinal pigmented epithelium. Proceedings of the National Academy of Sciences of the United States of America. 2014;**111**:8518-8523. DOI: 10.1073/pnas.1324212111

[42] Phillips MJ, Wallace KA, Dickerson SJ, Miller MJ, Verhoeven AD, Martin JM, et al. Blood-derived human iPS cells generate optic vesicle-like structures with the capacity to form retinal laminae and develop synapses. Investigative Ophthalmology & Visual Science. 2012;**53**:2007-2019. DOI: 10.1167/iovs.11-9313

[43] Lowe A, Harris R, Bhansali P, Cvekl A, Liu W. Intercellular adhesion-dependent

cell survival and ROCK-regulated Actomyosin-driven forces mediate self-formation of a retinal organoid. Stem Cell Reports. 2016;**6**:743-756. DOI: 10.1016/j.stemcr.2016.03.011

[44] Gonzalez-Cordero A, Kruczek K, Naeem A, Fernando M, Kloc M, Ribeiro J, et al. Recapitulation of human retinal development from human pluripotent stem cells generates transplantable populations of cone photoreceptors. Stem Cell Reports. 2017;**9**:820-837. DOI: 10.1016/j.stemcr.2017.07.022

[45] Kim S, Lowe A, Dharmat R, Lee S, Owen LA, Wang J, et al. Generation, transcriptome profiling, and functional validation of cone-rich human retinal organoids. Proceedings of the National Academy of Sciences of the United States of America. 2019;**116**:10824-10833. DOI: 10.1073/pnas.1901572116

[46] Rabesandratana O, Chaffiol A, Mialot A, Slembrouck-Brec A, Joffrois C, Nanteau C, et al. Generation of a transplantable population of human iPSC-derived retinal ganglion cells. Frontiers in Cell and Development Biology. 2020;**8**:585675. DOI: 10.3389/fcell.2020.585675

[47] Zhang X, Wang W, Jin ZB. Retinal organoids as models for development and diseases. Cell Regeneration. 2021;**10**:33. DOI: 10.1186/s13619-021-00097-1

[48] Chen HY, Kaya KD, Dong L, Swaroop A. Three-dimensional retinal organoids from mouse pluripotent stem cells mimic in vivo development with enhanced stratification and rod photoreceptor differentiation. Molecular Vision. 2016;**22**:1077

[49] Gao L, Chen X, Zeng Y, Li Q, Zou T, Chen S, et al. Intermittent high oxygen influences the formation of neural retinal tissue from human embryonic stem cells. Scientific Reports. 2016;**6**:29944. DOI: 10.1038/srep29944

[50] Akhtar T, Xie H, Khan MI, Zhao H, Bao J, Zhang M, et al. Accelerated photoreceptor differentiation of hiPSC-derived retinal organoids by contact co-culture with retinal pigment epithelium. Stem Cell Research. 2019;**39**:101491. DOI: 10.1016/j.scr.2019.101491

[51] Fligor CM, Lavekar SS, Harkin J, Shields PK, VanderWall KB, Huang KC, et al. Extension of retinofugal projections in an assembled model of human pluripotent stem cell-derived organoids. Stem Cell Reports. 2021;**16**:2228-2241. DOI: 10.1016/j.stemcr.2021.05.009

[52] Gabriel E, Albanna W, Pasquini G, Ramani A, Josipovic N, Mariappan A, et al. Human brain organoids assemble functionally integrated bilateral optic vesicles. Cell Stem Cell. 2021;**28**(1740-1757):e1748. DOI: 10.1016/j.stem.2021.07.010

[53] Luo Z, Zhong X, Li K, Xie B, Liu Y, Ye M, et al. An optimized system for effective derivation of three-dimensional retinal tissue via Wnt signaling regulation. Stem Cells. 2018;**36**:1709-1722. DOI: 10.1002/stem.2890

[54] Mellough CB, Collin J, Khazim M, White K, Sernagor E, Steel DH, et al. IGF-1 signaling plays an important role in the formation of three-dimensional laminated neural retina and other ocular structures from human embryonic stem cells. Stem Cells. 2015;**33**:2416-2430. DOI: 10.1002/stem.2023

[55] Zerti D, Molina MM, Dorgau B, Mearns S, Bauer R, Al-Aama J, et al. IGFBPs mediate IGF-1's functions in retinal lamination and photoreceptor development during pluripotent stem cell differentiation to retinal organoids. Stem

Cells. 2021;**39**:458-466. DOI: 10.1002/stem.3331

[56] Brooks MJ, Chen HY, Kelley RA, Mondal AK, Nagashima K, De Val N, et al. Improved retinal organoid differentiation by modulating signaling pathways revealed by comparative transcriptome analyses with development In vivo. Stem Cell Reports. 2019;**13**:891-905. DOI: 10.1016/j.stemcr.2019.09.009

[57] Ueda K, Onishi A, Ito SI, Nakamura M, Takahashi M. Generation of three-dimensional retinal organoids expressing rhodopsin and S- and M-cone opsins from mouse stem cells. Biochemical and Biophysical Research Communications. 2018;**495**:2595-2601. DOI: 10.1016/j.bbrc.2017.12.092

[58] Kaya KD, Chen HY, Brooks MJ, Kelley RA, Shimada H, Nagashima K, et al. Transcriptome-based molecular staging of human stem cell-derived retinal organoids uncovers accelerated photoreceptor differentiation by 9-cis retinal. Molecular Vision. 2019;**25**:663

[59] Pan D, Xia XX, Zhou H, Jin SQ, Lu YY, Liu H, et al. COCO enhances the efficiency of photoreceptor precursor differentiation in early human embryonic stem cell-derived retinal organoids. Stem Cell Research & Therapy. 2020;**11**:366. DOI: 10.1186/s13287-020-01883-5

[60] Zhang X, Jin ZB. Directed induction of retinal organoids from human pluripotent stem cells. Journal of Visualized Experiments. 2021;**170**:e62298. DOI: 10.3791/62298

[61] Eldred KC, Hadyniak SE, Hussey KA, Brenerman B, Zhang PW, Chamling X, et al. Thyroid hormone signaling specifies cone subtypes in human retinal organoids. Science. 2018;**362**:eaau6348. DOI: 10.1126/science.aau6348

[62] Ovando-Roche P, West EL, Branch MJ, Sampson RD, Fernando M, Munro P, et al. Use of bioreactors for culturing human retinal organoids improves photoreceptor yields. Stem Cell Research & Therapy. 2018;**9**:156. DOI: 10.1186/s13287-018-0907-0

[63] DiStefano T, Chen HY, Panebianco C, Kaya KD, Brooks MJ, Gieser L, et al. Accelerated and improved differentiation of retinal organoids from pluripotent stem cells in Rotating-Wall vessel bioreactors. Stem Cell Reports. 2018;**10**:300-313. DOI: 10.1016/j.stemcr.2017.11.001

[64] Singh D, Wang SB, Xia T, Tainsh L, Ghiassi-Nejad M, Xu T, et al. A biodegradable scaffold enhances differentiation of embryonic stem cells into a thick sheet of retinal cells. Biomaterials. 2018;**154**:158-168. DOI: 10.1016/j.biomaterials.2017.10.052

[65] Achberger K, Probst C, Haderspeck J, Bolz S, Rogal J, Chuchuy J, et al. Merging organoid and organ-on-a-chip technology to generate complex multi-layer tissue models in a human retina-on-a-chip platform. eLife. 2019;**8**:e46188. DOI: 10.7554/eLife.46188

[66] Decembrini S, Hoehnel S, Brandenberg N, Arsenijevic Y, Lutolf MP. Hydrogel-based milliwell arrays for standardized and scalable retinal organoid cultures. Scientific Reports. 2020;**10**:1-10. DOI: 10.1038/s41598-020-67012-7

[67] Xue Y, Seiler MJ, Tang WC, Wang JY, Delgado J, McLelland BT, et al. Retinal organoids on-a-chip: A micro-millifluidic bioreactor for long-term organoid maintenance. Lab on a Chip. 2021;**21**:3361-3377. DOI: 10.1039/d1lc00011j

[68] Eldred MK, Charlton-Perkins M, Muresan L, Harris WA. Self-organising

aggregates of zebrafish retinal cells for investigating mechanisms of neural lamination. Development. 2017;**144**:1097-1106. DOI: 10.1242/dev.142760

[69] Reichman S, Slembrouck A, Gagliardi G, Chaffiol A, Terray A, Nanteau C, et al. Generation of storable retinal organoids and retinal pigmented epithelium from adherent human iPS cells in Xeno-free and feeder-free conditions. Stem Cells. 2017;**35**:1176-1188. DOI: 10.1002/stem.2586

[70] Kobayashi W, Onishi A, Tu HY, Takihara Y, Matsumura M, Tsujimoto K, et al. Culture Systems of Dissociated Mouse and Human Pluripotent Stem Cell-Derived Retinal Ganglion Cells Purified by two-step Immunopanning. Investigative Ophthalmology & Visual Science. 2018;**59**:776-787. DOI: 10.1167/iovs.17-22406

[71] Zilova L, Weinhardt V, Tavhelidse T, Schlagheck C, Thumberger T, Wittbrodt J. Fish primary embryonic pluripotent cells assemble into retinal tissue mirroring in vivo early eye development. eLife. 2021;**10**. DOI: 10.7554/eLife.66998

[72] Buskin A, Zhu L, Chichagova V, Basu B, Mozaffari-Jovin S, Dolan D, et al. Disrupted alternative splicing for genes implicated in splicing and ciliogenesis causes PRPF31 retinitis pigmentosa. Nature Communications. 2018;**9**:4234. DOI: 10.1038/s41467-018-06448-y

[73] Deng WL, Gao ML, Lei XL, Lv JN, Zhao H, He KW, et al. Gene correction reverses ciliopathy and photoreceptor loss in iPSC-derived retinal organoids from retinitis Pigmentosa patients. Stem Cell Reports. 2018;**10**:1267-1281. DOI: 10.1016/j.stemcr.2018.02.003

[74] de Bruijn SE, Fiorentino A, Ottaviani D, Fanucchi S, Melo US, Corral-Serrano JC, et al. Structural variants create new topological-associated domains and ectopic retinal enhancer-gene contact in dominant retinitis Pigmentosa. The American Journal of Human Genetics. 2020;**107**:802-814. DOI: 10.1016/j.ajhg.2020.09.002

[75] Guo Y, Wang P, Ma JH, Cui Z, Yu Q, Liu S, et al. Modeling retinitis Pigmentosa: Retinal organoids generated from the iPSCs of a patient with the USH2A mutation show early developmental abnormalitics. Frontiers in Cellular Neuroscience. 2019;**13**:361. DOI: 10.3389/fncel.2019.00361

[76] Quinn PM, Buck TM, Mulder AA, Ohonin C, Alves CH, Vos RM, et al. Human iPSC-derived retinas recapitulate the fetal CRB1 CRB2 complex formation and demonstrate that photoreceptors and Muller glia are targets of AAV5. Stem Cell Reports. 2019;**12**:906-919. DOI: 10.1016/j.stemcr.2019.03.002

[77] Gao ML, Lei XL, Han F, He KW, Jin SQ, Zhang YY, et al. Patient-specific retinal organoids recapitulate disease features of late-onset retinitis Pigmentosa. Frontiers in Cell and Development Biology. 2020;**8**:128. DOI: 10.3389/fcell.2020.00128

[78] Sharma TP, Wiley LA, Whitmore SS, Anfinson KR, Cranston CM, Oppedal DJ, et al. Patient-specific induced pluripotent stem cells to evaluate the pathophysiology of TRNT1-associated retinitis pigmentosa. Stem Cell Research. 2017;**21**:58-70. DOI: 10.1016/j.scr.2017.03.005

[79] Tucker BA, Mullins RF, Streb LM, Anfinson K, Eyestone ME, Kaalberg E, et al. Patient-specific iPSC-derived photoreceptor precursor cells as a means to investigate retinitis pigmentosa. eLife. 2013;**2**:e00824. DOI: 10.7554/eLife.00824

[80] Arno G, Agrawal SA, Eblimit A, Bellingham J, Xu M, Wang F, et al. Mutations in REEP6 cause autosomal-recessive retinitis Pigmentosa. American Journal of Human Genetics. 2016;**99**:1305-1315. DOI: 10.1016/j.ajhg.2016.10.008

[81] Lane A, Jovanovic K, Shortall C, Ottaviani D, Panes AB, Schwarz N, et al. Modeling and rescue of RP2 retinitis Pigmentosa using iPSC-derived retinal organoids. Stem Cell Reports. 2020;**15**:67-79. DOI: 10.1016/j.stemcr.2020.05.007

[82] Kruczek K, Qu Z, Gentry J, Fadl BR, Gieser L, Hiriyanna S, et al. Gene therapy of dominant CRX-Leber congenital Amaurosis using patient stem cell-derived retinal organoids. Stem Cell Reports. 2021;**16**:252-263. DOI: 10.1016/j.stemcr.2020.12.018

[83] Li G, Gao G, Wang P, Song X, Xu P, Xie B, et al. Generation and characterization of induced pluripotent stem cells and retinal organoids from a Leber's congenital Amaurosis patient with novel RPE65 mutations. Frontiers in Molecular Neuroscience. 2019;**12**:212. DOI: 10.3389/fnmol.2019.00212

[84] Lukovic D, Artero Castro A, Kaya KD, Munezero D, Gieser L, Davo-Martinez C, et al. Retinal organoids derived from hiPSCs of an AIPL1-LCA patient maintain Cytoarchitecture despite reduced levels of mutant AIPL1. Scientific Reports. 2020;**10**:5426. DOI: 10.1038/s41598-020-62047-2

[85] Shimada H, Lu Q, Insinna-Kettenhofen C, Nagashima K, English MA, Semler EM, et al. In vitro modeling using ciliopathy-patient-derived cells reveals distinct cilia dysfunctions caused by CEP290 mutations. Cell Reports. 2017;**20**:384-396. DOI: 10.1016/j.celrep.2017.06.045

[86] Parfitt DA, Lane A, Ramsden CM, Carr AF, Munro PM, Jovanovic K, et al. Identification and correction of mechanisms underlying inherited blindness in human iPSC-derived optic cups. Cell Stem Cell. 2016;**18**:769-781. DOI: 10.1016/j.stem.2016.03.021

[87] Chirco KR, Chew S, Moore AT, Duncan JL, Lamba DA. Allele-specific gene editing to rescue dominant CRX-associated LCA7 phenotypes in a retinal organoid model. Stem Cell Reports. 2021;**16**:2690-2702. DOI: 10.1016/j.stemcr.2021.09.007

[88] Dulla K, Aguila M, Lane A, Jovanovic K, Parfitt DA, Schulkens I, et al. Splice-modulating oligonucleotide QR-110 restores CEP290 mRNA and function in human c.2991+1655A>G LCA10 models. Molecular Therapy Nucleic Acids. 2018;**12**:730-740. DOI: 10.1016/j.omtn.2018.07.010

[89] Deng X, Iwagawa T, Fukushima M, Watanabe S. Characterization of human-induced pluripotent stem cells carrying homozygous RB1 gene deletion. Genes to Cells. 2020;**25**:510-517. DOI: 10.1111/gtc.12771

[90] Liu H, Zhang Y, Zhang YY, Li YP, Hua ZQ, Zhang CJ, et al. Human embryonic stem cell-derived organoid retinoblastoma reveals a cancerous origin. Proceedings of the National Academy of Sciences of the United States of America. 2020;**117**:33628-33638. DOI: 10.1073/pnas.2011780117

[91] Norrie JL, Nityanandam A, Lai K, Chen X, Wilson M, Stewart E, et al. Retinoblastoma from human stem cell-derived retinal organoids. Nature Communications. 2021;**12**:4535. DOI: 10.1038/s41467-021-24781-7

[92] Kallman A, Capowski EE, Wang J, Kaushik AM, Jansen AD, Edwards KL,

et al. Investigating cone photoreceptor development using patient-derived NRL null retinal organoids. Communications Biology. 2020;**3**:82. DOI: 10.1038/s42003-020-0808-5

[93] Zhang X, Thompson JA, Zhang D, Charng J, Arunachalam S, McLaren TL, et al. Characterization of CRB1 splicing in retinal organoids derived from a patient with adult-onset rod-cone dystrophy caused by the c.1892A>G and c.2548G>A variants. Molecular Genetics & Genomic Medicine. 2020;**8**:e1489. DOI: 10.1002/mgg3.1489

[94] Gantner ML, Eade K, Wallace M, Handzlik MK, Fallon R, Trombley J, et al. Serine and lipid metabolism in macular disease and peripheral neuropathy. The New England Journal of Medicine. 2019;**381**:1422-1433. DOI: 10.1056/NEJMoa1815111

[95] Phillips MJ, Perez ET, Martin JM, Reshel ST, Wallace KA, Capowski EE, et al. Modeling human retinal development with patient-specific induced pluripotent stem cells reveals multiple roles for visual system homeobox 2. Stem Cells. 2014;**32**: 1480-1492. DOI: 10.1002/stem.1667

[96] Khan M, Arno G, Fakin A, Parfitt DA, Dhooge PPA, Albert S, et al. Detailed phenotyping and therapeutic strategies for Intronic ABCA4 variants in Stargardt disease. Molecular Therapy Nucleic Acids. 2020;**21**:412-427. DOI: 10.1016/j.omtn.2020.06.007

[97] Huang KC, Wang ML, Chen SJ, Kuo JC, Wang WJ, Nhi Nguyen PN, et al. Morphological and molecular defects in human three-dimensional retinal organoid model of X-linked juvenile Retinoschisis. Stem Cell Reports. 2019;**13**:906-923. DOI: 10.1016/j.stemcr.2019.09.010

[98] Zhang XH, Jin ZB. Patient iPSC-derived retinal organoids: Observable retinal diseases in-a-dish. Histology and Histopathology. 2021;**36**:705-710. DOI: 10.14670/HH-18-307

[99] Ran X, Cai WJ, Huang XF, Liu Q, Lu F, Qu J, et al. 'RetinoGenetics': A comprehensive mutation database for genes related to inherited retinal degeneration. Database: The Journal of Biological Databases and Curation. 2014;**2014**. DOI: 10.1093/database/bau047

[100] Tsang SH, Sharma T. Leber congenital Amaurosis. In: Tsang SH, Sharma T, editors. Atlas of Inherited Retinal Diseases. Cham: Springer International Publishing; 2018. pp. 131-137

[101] Li YP, Deng WL, Jin ZB. Modeling retinitis pigmentosa through patient-derived retinal organoids. STAR Protocols. 2021;**2**:100438. DOI: 10.1016/j.xpro.2021.100438

[102] Dimaras H, Kimani K, Dimba EA, Gronsdahl P, White A, Chan HS, et al. Retinoblastoma. The Lancet. 2012;**379**:1436-1446

[103] Friend SH, Bernards R, Rogelj S, Weinberg RA, Rapaport JM, Albert DM, et al. A human DNA segment with properties of the gene that predisposes to retinoblastoma and osteosarcoma. Nature. 1986;**323**:643-646

[104] Liu H, Hua ZQ, Jin ZB. Modeling human retinoblastoma using embryonic stem cell-derived retinal organoids. STAR Protocols. 2021;**2**:100444. DOI: 10.1016/j.xpro.2021.100444

[105] Zhang X, Zhang D, Thompson JA, Chen SC, Huang Z, Jennings L, et al. Gene correction of the CLN3 c.175G>a variant in patient-derived induced pluripotent stem cells prevents pathological changes in retinal organoids.

Molecular Genetics & Genomic Medicine. 2021;**9**:e1601. DOI: 10.1002/mgg3.1601

[106] Diakatou M, Dubois G, Erkilic N, Sanjurjo-Soriano C, Meunier I, Kalatzis V. Allele-specific knockout by CRISPR/Cas to treat autosomal dominant retinitis Pigmentosa caused by the G56R mutation in NR2E3. International Journal of Molecular Sciences. 2021;**22**:2607. DOI: 10.3390/ijms22052607

[107] Russell S, Bennett J, Wellman JA, Chung DC, Yu Z-F, Tillman A, et al. Efficacy and safety of voretigene neparvovec (AAV2-hRPE65v2) in patients with RPE65-mediated inherited retinal dystrophy: A randomised, controlled, open-label, phase 3 trial. The Lancet. 2017;**390**:849-860. DOI: 10.1016/s0140-6736(17)31868-8

[108] Mookherjee S, Chen HY, Isgrig K, Yu W, Hiriyanna S, Levron R, et al. A CEP290 C-terminal domain complements the mutant CEP290 of Rd16 mice In trans and rescues retinal degeneration. Cell Reports. 2018;**25**(611-623):e616. DOI: 10.1016/j.celrep.2018.09.043

[109] MacLaren RE, Pearson RA, MacNeil A, Douglas RH, Salt TE, Akimoto M, et al. Retinal repair by transplantation of photoreceptor precursors. Nature. 2006;**444**:203-207. DOI: 10.1038/nature05161

[110] Bartsch U, Oriyakhel W, Kenna PF, Linke S, Richard G, Petrowitz B, et al. Retinal cells integrate into the outer nuclear layer and differentiate into mature photoreceptors after subretinal transplantation into adult mice. Experimental Eye Research. 2008;**86**:691-700. DOI: 10.1016/j.exer.2008.01.018

[111] Lakowski J, Baron M, Bainbridge J, Barber AC, Pearson RA, Ali RR, et al. Cone and rod photoreceptor transplantation in models of the childhood retinopathy Leber congenital amaurosis using flow-sorted Crx-positive donor cells. Human Molecular Genetics. 2010;**19**:4545-4559. DOI: 10.1093/hmg/ddq378

[112] Eberle D, Schubert S, Postel K, Corbeil D, Ader M. Increased integration of transplanted CD73-positive photoreceptor precursors into adult mouse retina. Investigative Ophthalmology & Visual Science. 2011;**52**:6462-6471. DOI: 10.1167/iovs.11-7399

[113] Pearson RA, Barber AC, Rizzi M, Hippert C, Xue T, West EL, et al. Restoration of vision after transplantation of photoreceptors. Nature. 2012;**485**:99-103. DOI: 10.1038/nature10997

[114] Barber AC, Hippert C, Duran Y, West EL, Bainbridge JW, Warre-Cornish K, et al. Repair of the degenerate retina by photoreceptor transplantation. Proceedings of the National Academy of Sciences of the United States of America. 2013;**110**:354-359. DOI: 10.1073/pnas.1212677110

[115] Singh MS, Charbel Issa P, Butler R, Martin C, Lipinski DM, Sekaran S, et al. Reversal of end-stage retinal degeneration and restoration of visual function by photoreceptor transplantation. Proceedings of the National Academy of Sciences of the United States of America. 2013;**110**:1101-1106. DOI: 10.1073/pnas.1119416110

[116] Lamba DA, Gust J, Reh TA. Transplantation of human embryonic stem cell-derived photoreceptors restores some visual function in Crx-deficient mice. Cell Stem Cell. 2009;**4**:73-79. DOI: 10.1016/j.stem.2008.10.015

[117] West EL, Gonzalez-Cordero A, Hippert C, Osakada F, Martinez-Barbera JP,

Pearson RA, et al. Defining the integration capacity of embryonic stem cell-derived photoreceptor precursors. Stem Cells. 2012;**30**:1424-1435. DOI: 10.1002/stem.1123

[118] Jin ZB, Gao ML, Deng WL, Wu KC, Sugita S, Mandai M, et al. Stemming retinal regeneration with pluripotent stem cells. Progress in Retinal and Eye Research. 2019;**69**:38-56. DOI: 10.1016/j.preteyeres.2018.11.003

[119] Gonzalez-Cordero A, West EL, Pearson RA, Duran Y, Carvalho LS, Chu CJ, et al. Photoreceptor precursors derived from three-dimensional embryonic stem cell cultures integrate and mature within adult degenerate retina. Nature Biotechnology. 2013;**31**:741-747. DOI: 10.1038/nbt.2643

[120] Decembrini S, Koch U, Radtke F, Moulin A, Arsenijevic Y. Derivation of traceable and transplantable photoreceptors from mouse embryonic stem cells. Stem Cell Reports. 2014;**2**:853-865. DOI: 10.1016/j.stemcr.2014.04.010

[121] Assawachananont J, Mandai M, Okamoto S, Yamada C, Eiraku M, Yonemura S, et al. Transplantation of embryonic and induced pluripotent stem cell-derived 3D retinal sheets into retinal degenerative mice. Stem Cell Reports. 2014;**2**:662-674. DOI: 10.1016/j.stemcr.2014.03.011

[122] Shirai H, Mandai M, Matsushita K, Kuwahara A, Yonemura S, Nakano T, et al. Transplantation of human embryonic stem cell-derived retinal tissue in two primate models of retinal degeneration. Proceedings of the National Academy of Sciences of the United States of America. 2016;**113**:E81-E90. DOI: 10.1073/pnas.1512590113

[123] Santos-Ferreira T, Volkner M, Borsch O, Haas J, Cimalla P, Vasudevan P, et al. Stem cell-derived photoreceptor transplants differentially integrate into mouse models of cone-rod dystrophy. Investigative Ophthalmology & Visual Science. 2016;**57**:3509-3520. DOI: 10.1167/iovs.16-19087

[124] Kruczek K, Gonzalez-Cordero A, Goh D, Naeem A, Jonikas M, Blackford SJI, et al. Differentiation and transplantation of embryonic stem cell-derived cone photoreceptors into a mouse model of end-stage retinal degeneration. Stem Cell Reports. 2017;**8**:1659-1674. DOI: 10.1016/j.stemcr.2017.04.030

[125] Zhu J, Reynolds J, Garcia T, Cifuentes H, Chew S, Zeng X, et al. Generation of transplantable retinal photoreceptors from a current good manufacturing practice-manufactured human induced pluripotent stem cell line. Stem Cells Translational Medicine. 2018;**7**:210-219. DOI: 10.1002/sctm.17-0205

[126] Iraha S, Tu HY, Yamasaki S, Kagawa T, Goto M, Takahashi R, et al. Establishment of Immunodeficient retinal degeneration model mice and functional maturation of human ESC-derived retinal sheets after transplantation. Stem Cell Reports. 2018;**10**:1059-1074. DOI: 10.1016/j.stemcr.2018.01.032

[127] McLelland BT, Lin B, Mathur A, Aramant RB, Thomas BB, Nistor G, et al. Transplanted hESC-derived retina organoid sheets differentiate, integrate, and improve visual function in retinal degenerate rats. Investigative Ophthalmology & Visual Science. 2018;**59**:2586-2603. DOI: 10.1167/iovs.17-23646

[128] Gagliardi G, Ben M'Barek K, Chaffiol A, Slembrouck-Brec A, Conart JB, Nanteau C, et al. Characterization and transplantation of CD73-positive photoreceptors

isolated from human iPSC-derived retinal organoids. Stem Cell Reports. 2018;**11**:665-680. DOI: 10.1016/j.stemcr.2018.07.005

[129] Collin J, Zerti D, Queen R, Santos-Ferreira T, Bauer R, Coxhead J, et al. CRX expression in pluripotent stem cell-derived photoreceptors Marks a transplantable subpopulation of early cones. Stem Cells. 2019;**37**:609-622. DOI: 10.1002/stem.2974

[130] Zou T, Gao L, Zeng Y, Li Q, Li Y, Chen S, et al. Organoid-derived C-kit (+)/SSEA4(−) human retinal progenitor cells promote a protective retinal microenvironment during transplantation in rodents. Nature Communications. 2019;**10**:1205. DOI: 10.1038/s41467-019-08961-0

[131] Garita-Hernandez M, Lampic M, Chaffiol A, Guibbal L, Routet F, Santos-Ferreira T, et al. Restoration of visual function by transplantation of optogenetically engineered photoreceptors. Nature Communications. 2019;**10**:4524. DOI: 10.1038/s41467-019-12330-2

[132] Eastlake K, Wang W, Jayaram H, Murray-Dunning C, Carr AJF, Ramsden CM, et al. Phenotypic and functional characterization of Muller glia isolated from induced pluripotent stem cell-derived retinal organoids: Improvement of retinal ganglion cell function upon transplantation. Stem Cells Translational Medicine. 2019;**8**: 775-784. DOI: 10.1002/sctm.18-0263

[133] Singh RK, Occelli LM, Binette F, Petersen-Jones SM, Nasonkin IO. Transplantation of human embryonic stem cell-derived retinal tissue in the subretinal space of the cat eye. Stem Cells and Development. 2019;**28**:1151-1166. DOI: 10.1089/scd.2019.0090

[134] Lin B, McLelland BT, Aramant RB, Thomas BB, Nistor G, Keirstead HS, et al. Retina organoid transplants develop photoreceptors and improve visual function in RCS rats with RPE dysfunction. Investigative Ophthalmology & Visual Science. 2020;**61**:34. DOI: 10.1167/iovs.61.11.34

[135] Ribeiro J, Procyk CA, West EL, O'Hara-Wright M, Martins MF, Khorasani MM, et al. Restoration of visual function in advanced disease after transplantation of purified human pluripotent stem cell-derived cone photoreceptors. Cell Reports. 2021;**35**:109022. DOI: 10.1016/j.celrep.2021.109022

[136] Luo Z, Xian B, Li K, Li K, Yang R, Chen M, et al. Biodegradable scaffolds facilitate epiretinal transplantation of hiPSC-derived retinal neurons in nonhuman primates. Acta Biomaterialia. 2021;**134**:289-301. DOI: 10.1016/j.actbio.2021.07.040

[137] He XY, Zhao CJ, Xu H, Chen K, Bian BS, Gong Y, et al. Synaptic repair and vision restoration in advanced degenerating eyes by transplantation of retinal progenitor cells. Stem Cell Reports. 2021;**16**:1805-1817. DOI: 10.1016/j.stemcr.2021.06.002

[138] Thomas BB, Lin B, Martinez-Camarillo JC, Zhu D, McLelland BT, Nistor G, et al. Co-grafts of human embryonic stem cell derived retina organoids and retinal pigment epithelium for retinal reconstruction in Immunodeficient retinal degenerate Royal College of surgeons rats. Frontiers in Neuroscience. 2021;**15**:752958. DOI: 10.3389/fnins.2021.752958

[139] Ito SI, Onishi A, Takahashi M. Chemically-induced photoreceptor degeneration and protection in mouse iPSC-derived three-dimensional

retinal organoids. Stem Cell Research. 2017;**24**:94-101. DOI: 10.1016/j.scr.2017.08.018

[140] Garita-Hernandez M, Guibbal L, Toualbi L, Routet F, Chaffiol A, Winckler C, et al. Optogenetic light sensors in human retinal organoids. Frontiers in Neuroscience. 2018;**12**:789. DOI: 10.3389/fnins.2018.00789

[141] Rathnasamy G, Foulds WS, Ling E-A, Kaur C. Retinal microglia—A key player in healthy and diseased retina. Progress in Neurobiology. 2019;**173**:18-40

[142] Mansour AA, Gonçalves JT, Bloyd CW, Li H, Fernandes S, Quang D, et al. An in vivo model of functional and vascularized human brain organoids. Nature Biotechnology. 2018;**36**:432-441

[143] Cakir B, Xiang Y, Tanaka Y, Kural MH, Parent M, Kang Y-J, et al. Engineering of human brain organoids with a functional vascular-like system. Nature Methods. 2019;**16**:1169-1175

[144] Richards D, Jia J, Yost M, Markwald R, Mei Y. 3D bioprinting for vascularized tissue fabrication. Annals of Biomedical Engineering. 2017;**45**:132-147. DOI: 10.1007/s10439-016-1653-z

[145] Worsdorfer P, Dalda N, Kern A, Kruger S, Wagner N, Kwok CK, et al. Generation of complex human organoid models including vascular networks by incorporation of mesodermal progenitor cells. Scientific Reports. 2019;**9**:15663. DOI: 10.1038/s41598-019-52204-7

Section 4

Organoid and Cancer

Chapter 5

Evolution of Organoids in Oncology

Allen Thayakumar Basanthakumar, Janitha Chandrasekhar Darlybai and Jyothsna Ganesh

Abstract

An organoid is an *in-vitro* platform that recreates 3D multicellular aggerates to form tissues that fabricate the human cellular environment in the lab and imitate the functionalities of the specific organ or disease. Organoids effectively overcomes the gaps in research between 2D cell line and *in-vivo* models. For organoid development, both pluripotent stem cells and embryonic stem cells can be utilized, and recently Patient-Derived Organoids (PDO) was developed that overcome the limitations caused by using other cell lines. With the development of many advanced technologies in the field of research, the organoid evolution also progressed slowly into the development of patient-specific organ structures. Since tumor organoids were heterogeneous as well as patient-specific, it has many advantages that aid cancer therapy effectively. Apart from cancer treatment, organoids have a variety of applications in cancer research, the study of tissue-specific models, and also in the analysis of the relationship between tissue-specific cancer with various pathogens. Thus, the development of organoids in an effective way can pave the way for various biomedical applications. This chapter focuses on the trends in the journey of organoid research and the latest technologies developed specifically for organoids.

Keywords: organoid, 3D tissues, cancer research, cancer therapy

1. Introduction

Cancer is a heterogeneous disease that is caused by the progress of somatic mutations in normal cells [1]. Based on studies it was confirmed that continuous exposure to physical agents such as X-rays, gamma rays, UV rays, and genotoxic factors may end up in the progress of cancer cells from normal cells [2]. Carcinogenesis is a complex process that involves various pathways which need to be studied to understand the response and treatment method required for targeted therapy which is a complicated mechanism [3].

The development of drugs by using medicinal plants as bio source has also been studied extensively in various research [4]. It is essential to understand the biological interaction among immune cells among tumor immune microenvironment, stroma, and tumor for the success of cancer clinical treatments [5]. The overall cancer therapy may vary with multiple metastatic sites which in turn depend on the tumor

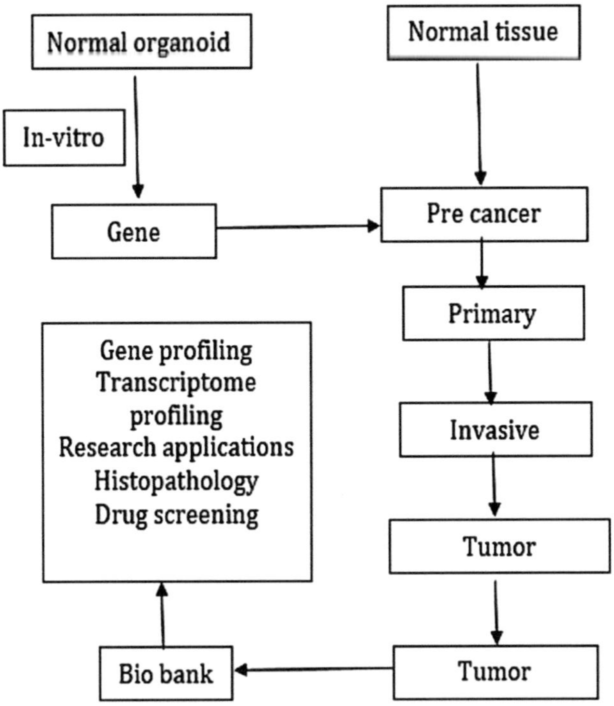

Figure 1.
Flowchart of use of normal organoids in making tumor organoids and utilization of tumor organoids in a biobank and its applications [13–18].

heterogeneity [6]. The major biological complexities make the treatment methods difficult which in turn varies with the metastatic sites among individual patients [7]. The microenvironment of tumor cells includes normal stroma, malignant cells, and immune response based on every individual [8]. The durability and patient-to-patient response extremely varies based on each patient and hence very difficult to predict the consequences [9].

An organoid is an emerging technology with various applications in biomedical applications such as biobanking, disease modeling, regenerative medicine, and precision medicine [10]. An organoid is a technology used to fabricate 3D tissues in the laboratory that resembles parent tissue in function and structure and hence bridges the gap between 2D *in-vitro* and *in-vivo* models so that they can be utilized effectively in cancer research [11]. Though many cancer treatments were available the tumor heterogeneity limits the treatment as the drug sensitivity, drug invasion ability, growth rate of tumor changes based on individuals [12]. In the current review, the history and progressions in the developments of organoids were elaborated accompanied by their applications in cancer treatment along with their limits and steps required to overcome the limitations so that the organoid technology can be implemented efficiently in future research. Overview showed in **Figure 1**.

2. The use of humanized models for cancer treatment

In the initial phase, the genetically engineered mouse models (GEMMs) provided a better appreciation for cancer treatment [19]. But later for practical applications,

GEMMs technologies were identified to be expensive, laborious, and fetch up into complications when transformed into therapeutic applications [20]. One of the methods of generation of organoids is the utilization of Pluripotent stem cells (iPSCs), but the tissues generated from these embryonic stem cells were found to be phenotypically unstable and hence have the same limitations [21]. Later, Patient-derived xenografts (PDXs) were contemplated as a better replacement to conquer these constraints since, in this technology, models were provoked from an enormous pool of patients [22]. Unfortunately, these techniques also ended up in complications as the cancer cell lines generated *in-vitro* were genetically unstable and were devoid of the cellular microenvironment of tumor cells *in-vivo* and in most cases these cell lines ended up in unmatched cell lines from normal tissue which was considered as control cell lines [23].

Patient-derived tumor xenografts (PDTXs) is the recently available technology in cancer research that can maintain genomic stability and tumor heterogeneity but the major drawback of PDXs is that it is expensive and time-consuming and hence treatment gets delayed [13]. Later PDTXs technologies were upgraded by transplanting these cell lines into mouse models, but PDTXs failed to replicate the human-specific immune systems and were also ended up as a laborious and expensive process [14]. The clinical response of cancer treatment depends on the clinical model used for the study [24].

3. Organoids and their types

The unique way to improve cancer research has emerged with the help of organoid technology that accompanies tumor heterogeneity at low cost and with less time [25]. Cancer organoids serve as an effective tool to understand the interaction between tumor environment and genetic alterations [15]. The organoids derived from postnatal or adult tissue were termed ASC-derived organoids. In the case of ESCs and iPSCs derived organoids, the generation of organoids takes place from all three germ layers. For all these types of organoids, the growth of cells was carried out by using a series of differentiation protocols by utilizing growth factors and inhibitors in the process of organogenesis [11]. Recently many patient-derived organoids (PDTOs) have been developed that include liver, prostate cancer, and pancreatic cancer organoids [26]. A snapshot of types is shown in **Figure 2**.

To make more clarity to organoids, CRISPER gene-editing technology is being implemented to organoid to convert normal organoids into tumor organoids [25]. Upon various research, mutations have been induced in normal organoids like intestinal organoids [40], colon organoids [41], pancreatic organoids [42] to make them into tumor organoids that paves the way for flexible *in-vitro* cancer models. Apart from carcinogenesis, cancer organoids were also being implemented to study cancer metastasis which is the process of spreading cancer cells to other parts of the body [43]. Cancer organoids have also extended their applications in drug screening since PDTOs can be utilized to study gene expression, pathology, and tissue-specific genetic alterations [44]. Few researchers have used cancer organoids to generate tumor-reactive T cells that can be used in immunotherapy [45].

The brief details about various types of organoids have been discussed below:

3.1 Intestinal organoids

The pluripotent stem cells (iPSCs) were used to derive intestinal organoids that contain both mesenchymal and epithelial cells [27]. The basic intestinal crypt cells

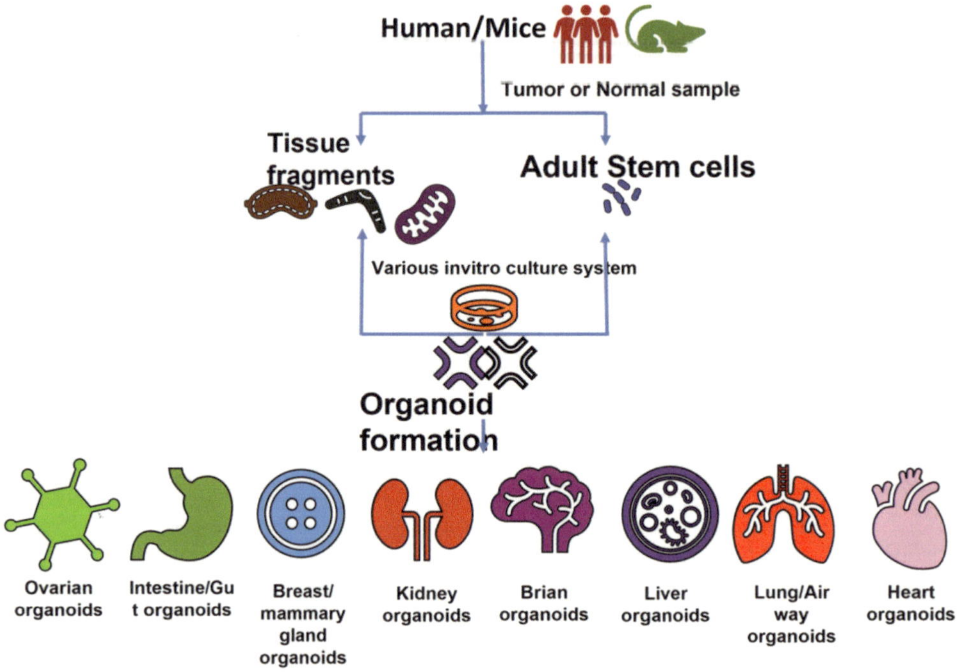

Figure 2.
Development of 3D organoids culture [27–39].

were allowed to grow in an appropriate medium containing a matrix that tends to organize into 3D epithelial cells that contain both physical and genetic resemblance of their parent organ [28].

3.2 Colon organoids

The colon organoids were originated from intestinal crypts in the presence of appropriate growth factors [29]. The stem cells of intestinal crypts differentiate into an epithelial complex that contains all types of intestinal cells. The isolated crypts develop into three-dimensional epithelial cells that form a sphere towards the lumen that further develops into colon organoids [30].

3.3 Pancreatic organoids

The capability of pancreatic ducts in in-vitro expansion and development of three-dimensional hollow structures in the presence of collagen as the suitable medium is utilized in the development of pancreatic organoids [31]. Many recent developments were carried out in establishing three-dimensional adult pancreatic organoids as well as fetal pancreatic organoids and both types of organoids were found to differ in morphology similar to that of parent cells [32].

3.4 Endometrial organoids

To investigate the biological processes involved in disease modeling, endometrial organoids were developed from primary endometrial cells of the human being [33]. For the development of three-dimensional endometrial organoids, the primary endometrial cells were dissociated, suspended in a Matrigel medium that promotes endometrial organ formation [34].

3.5 Lung organoids

The lung organoids were developed from stem cells of the lungs through a self-organization process [35–37]. The lung organoid technology has also been extended to develop various structures of lungs such as lung buds, airways, and alveolar cells that can be used to treat pulmonary diseases [38].

3.6 Ovarian organoids

Ovarian cancer is spread among a wide range of populations and the development of patient-specific ovarian organoids was found to be one of the precise approaches to enhance the treatment of ovarian cancer [39]. The ovarian organoid can enumerate the morphological heterogeneity of parent tissue and can aid in personalized therapy to enhance the treatment efficiency [46].

3.7 Breast organoids

Breast cancer is considered to be one of the most widely spread cancers among women with various subtypes and more heterogeneity [47]. Many studies have been performed on breast organoids and breast organoids can be grown either from epithelial cells [48] or from adult stem cells (ASCs) [27].

3.8 Retinal organoids

Retinal organoids were developed from Human Pluripotent Stem Cells (hPSCs) that is considered a labor-intensive and simple method of organoid development [49]. The retinal organoids also developed a physiological response to light to a certain extent that can be used in certain therapies [50].

3.9 Heart organoids

The heart organoids have proven to exhibit structural and functional features of developing human hearts [51]. The human Pluripotent Stem Cells (hPSCs) were used to develop in-vitro cardiac cell types that help in understanding and treatment of various cardiac diseases [52].

3.10 Brain organoids

The summons besotted in understanding the diseases caused in the central nervous system has been overcome by the development of brain organoids from either human Pluripotent Stem Cells (hPSCs) or epithelial cells [53].

4. Advantages of organoids over 2D techniques for cancer treatment

The development of organoid technology has overcome the limitations caused by 2D cell cultures in the following ways: 2D cultures were not repetitive of parent cultures while organoids were a portrait of their parent cells, the lack of predictivity faced in the use of 2D cultures was not visible while using organoid technology, and in 2D cell, culture models waste were being generated from growth medium which was overcome by organoid technology [54]. In organoid technology, multiple cell types were developed *in-vivo* that resemble the parent cells that have enormous applications in cancer research [11]. Tumor modeling is one of the vital applications of organoids as this technology help in identifying toxicity and effect of drugs before administering to patients which is not possible in 2D technology [40]. Organoids have strengthened the understanding of various disease progression and also helped scientists to study the pathways of disease carefully that enhance the treatment methods [55]. Organoids have extended their applications in various fields such as fundamental research [56], disease modeling [57], development of personalized medicine [58], and transplantation [59].

To overcome the technological limitations of cancer treatment, organoids were developed in which ASCs were proliferated in-vitro and self-organized into 3D structures by utilizing extracellular matrix proteins like BME and Matrigel as medium [60]. The main advantage of organoid technology is tissue-specific growth factors can be utilized based on the epithelial cells used for analysis [61]. Based on numerous studies, the ASCs derived organoids were found to be genetically and phenotypically stable and permit the expansion of stem cells in a required path which allows them to differentiate into tissue-specific cells [62]. Apart from tumor heterogeneity, more focus is required on lymphocyte infiltration trafficking along with the clinical response of individual patients to cancer treatment [63].

5. Stages of organoid development

Generally, the 3D culture of organoids was performed by using Matrigel derived from EHS (Engelbreth-Holam-Swarm) mouse sarcoma cells which were rich in adhesive proteins such as laminin, entactin, collagen, and proteoglycans. The Matrigel structural support, ECM signals along with the extracellular environment that supports the growth of cells [64]. In other techniques, Matrigel or fibroblasts were submerged in a medium to expose the upper layers of cells in the air. Later, the air-liquid interface will be utilized to culture the cells for better polarization and differentiation [65]. The organoid technology developed drastically after the successful generation of in-vitro organ generation from sponge cells [66], amphibians pronephros [67], chick embryos [68] followed by surface adhesion of cells using thermodynamic differentiation [69]. After the invention of pluripotent stem cells from mouse embryos, there was a significant impact on organoid development by utilizing stem cells [70].

The use of animal models has been considered in the initial days to predict the efficacy of drugs to tumor cells, later cell lines cultured in-vitro were used. But both these studies did not represent the actual model of tumor cells for which treatment is required [19]. A report by Radhakrishnan et al., 2017 [71] was used to analyze the immune target therapy for the treatment of cancer was carried out by utilizing the CANscript exvivo platform technology.

The various stages of organoid development were explained below [72] and the overview showed in **Figure 3**.

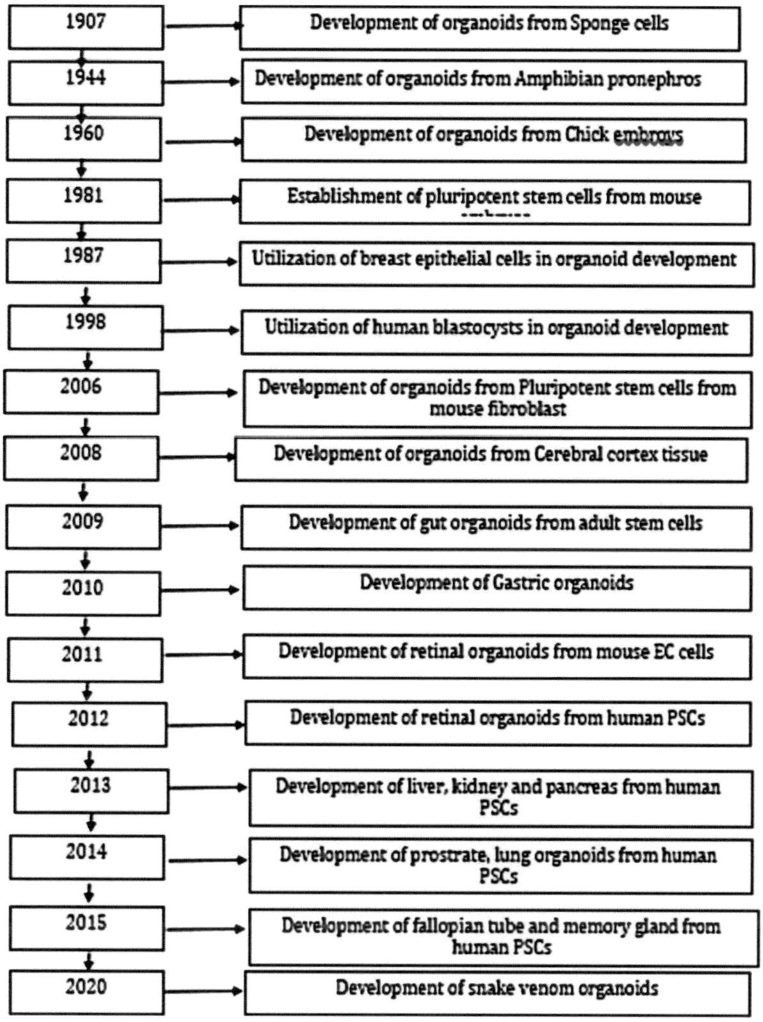

Figure 3.
Flowchart of various stages of organoid development [10, 19].

- 1900–1950: In the early 1900s hanging drop culture method was employed in organ development followed by tube cultures. Subsequently in 1907 organoids were developed from sponge cells and later in 1944 organoid development was carried out from amphibian pronephros.

- 1950–1980: In 1952 organoids were developed from chick embryos. In 1975 floating collagen cells were developed followed by characterization of laminin using organoid technology in 1979.

- 1980–2000: The isolation of pluripotent stem cells from mouse tails was successfully performed in 1981 which paved the way for great progress in organoid technology in subsequent years. The development of human blastocytes was performed in 1998.

- 2000–2020: The development of the first organoid from pluripotent stem cells was performed in 2006 from mouse fibroblast, followed by the development of organoids from cortex tissue, adult stem cells, development of gastric organoids, development of retinal, kidney, pancreas, lungs, fallopian tubes and snake venom were performed successfully in subsequent years.

6. Role of organoids in drug development and cancer research

Apart from therapeutic applications, organoids can also be employed in cancer research to study the mechanism of cancer progression and the interaction between pathogens and organs in the development of cancer cells. In a study conducted by Scanu et al., 2016 [73] the interaction of pathogen *Salmonella enterica* with the gall bladder cells was found to provoke gall bladder carcinoma. Similarly, in a study conducted by Yin et al., 2015 [74] relations between hepatic virus and liver cell carcinoma have been studied extensively.

Organoid technology has also been implemented to study the genetic interaction between mutation and progression of various types of cancer [75]. Organoids guide in the study of the initiation of tumors with the progression of cancer at various genetic levels [76].

Organoids can be used to study the response of drugs to each patient so can be utilized in drug development for cancer research [77]. Though many drugs were working on cancer models they get eliminated in final clinical trials due to unbearable side effects or lack of efficiency compared to clinical models [78]. Many biobanks of organoids were used to study the efficiency of novel drugs [16]. By utilizing organoids in drug screening, it will be feasible to predict the patient's response and value of Patient-Derived Organoids in chemotherapy. The data obtained from PDOs can be used to predict the outcome of individual patients which was not possible by using the cell line technique [17].

7. The use of biobanks for organoid research

The progression on the development of organoids from ASCs paved the way for the establishment of the biobank for cancer [18]. The cancer biobanks provide cancer organoid cultures of numerous cancer subtypes [79]. Based on an investigation of numerous organoids using biobanks it was concluded that the dependency of organoids on ligands varies from one type of organoids to other types of organoids [59]. The inception of biobanks of organoids for cancer paved the way for the up-gradation of anti-cancer drugs with a wide range of testing based on requirements by cancer patients [21]. In a study done by Smalley and coworkers in 2018 [80], CD 34 biomarker has been utilized effectively in cancer treatment and the outcome has been studied in detail.

8. Technological developments of organoids

The existing *in-vitro* and *in-vivo* platforms used for cancer therapy were proved to be not much effective and hence there is a need to derive many new platforms for cancer treatment [81]. In a study conducted by Majumder et al., 2015 [82], an attempt has been carried out to overcome the tumor heterogeneity with the help of the CANScriptTM platform designed by their team. In 2013, Radhakrishnana and his coworkers [83] attempted to design a drug PAT-1102 that acts as a HDAC (Histone deacetylase) inhibitor and hence can be utilized for cancer treatment. The utilization of Light-screening fluorescence microscopy, confocal microscopy, and multiphoton laser screening microscopy in organoid development can be used to visualize the 3D image of polarized and nonpolarized cells based on the individual organoid model [84]. Organoids have been utilized effectively to understand human brain development and also about various diseases elaborately [85]. Apart from cancer research organoids were also used to study various infectious diseases [86], genetic diseases by combing with CRISPER technology [87], to study the gene function [88] and cell development [89].

The development of organoids paved the way for 3D imaging technology which can be used to visualize complex organizations that were not possible using 2D imaging technology [90]. The 3D imaging technology helped scientists to visualize cellular components, intracellular processes, and architecture of cells in a detailed manner [91]. Lungs were considered as one of the most complex organs in the human body with numerous types of cells and the development of lung organoids had a significant impact on the treatment of lung cancer, asthma, cystic fibrosis, and pulmonary fibrosis [92]. Based on 3D imaging technology major therapeutic drugs were developed that can be used successfully in lung cancer treatment [93]. The 3D models increased the predictability and reliability of preclinical assays and decreased the use of animal models [94]. The quantitative analysis of the organization of various cell types in aggregates uses 3D imaging technology for detailed analysis [95].

Another technological up-gradation seen in organoid technology is Organs-on-a-chip which is used to model various functional groups of organs for detailed study [96]. Initially, the anatomy of the particular organ was studied, and then its basic elements were investigated that can be used to study organ-specific physical and biochemical applications [97]. Retinal diseases were one of the major causes of vision loss in humans worldwide while the complexity of neuro-retinal organization and complex blood supply causes side effects by the use of therapeutic drugs in the treatment of retinal diseases [98]. The development of retinal organoids improved the treatment methods of retinal diseases and also organs-on-a-chip technology paved the way to study cell types in detail that can further enhance the treatment methodology of retinal disease [99]. In case the focus of cancer research is based on a particular cell type or organ miniature types of organoids can be developed by utilizing organ-on-a-chip technology [100]. The organoid development and organoid-on-a-chip technology has their unique characteristics and limitations and based on research requirement the suitable technology is to be utilized [101]. The usage of organoid-on-a-chip technology on brain organoids paved the way to cure many neurological diseases [102].

In earlier days, tumor spheroids were developed to analyze the capability of antitumor therapeutic drugs, and recently tissue-specific organoids were utilized effectively to model various organs that can be used in cancer treatment by overcoming the limitations of ethical concerns caused by tumor spheroids [103]. The use of brain organoids to study neural diseases has proven that the brain organoids developed in 3D cultures express a large number of genes entangled in neurological problems and hence make the study process feasible compared to 2D technology [104]. In recent areas of research organoid technology is being implemented extensively in image-based phenotypic high throughput screening [105].

9. Limitations of organoids

Generation of organoids from epithelial cells may lead to contamination or overgrowth of normal cells [58]. Generally, the organoids developed from cancer cells will have less growth than organoids developed from normal cells which result in overgrowth of normal cells in the medium which can be overcome by limiting the use of growth factors in the medium [106]. Upon analyzing the efficiency of various organoids on drug development in-vitro, a positive predictive value of 88% and a negative predictive value of 100% were endorsed upon numerous studies [107, 108]. The organoids developed *in-vitro* lack the native microenvironment like stromal cells, immune cells [109]. This limitation can be overcome by culturing the tissues with required cellular elements for proper differentiation but this may end up in more cost [110]. In a study by [111], a high-throughput screening accompanied with patient-derived 3D organoids has been successfully utilized to overcome the limitations of organoids in drug screening. In another study, an organ-on-a-chip platform has been devised which contains hollow microchannels filled with living cells resembling human organs and organoids which can be utilized effectively for drug screening [112]. Another major limitation in organoid development is lack of reproducibility, laborious and costly method [113].

10. Conclusions

Cancer is a heterogeneous disease caused by a mutation in normal cells that results in the abnormal growth of cells. Though many treatment methods and drugs were available in cancer treatment, there is no proper cure, and the drugs used ended up in major side effects in patients. The development of cancer cells varies with the patient and also based on the type of cancer. Thus, there was a need to derive a patient-specific treatment method is cancer treatment. But the limitation of these 2D cell line models where it was a time-consuming process, expensive, and sometimes cannot meet the requirement of tumor heterogeneity to large extent. To overcome this many technologies such as GEMMs and PDTXs were developed and they have been proved to be effective techniques. To overcome these limitations organoid technology has emerged in which tissues were grown in *in-vitro* from cells derived from patients and these tissues can be utilized for drug development. Apart from drug development in cancer research organoid technology also paved the way to study elaborately the mechanisms behind cancer treatment, about particular organs in detail, and also the relationship between pathogens and various types of cancer. The culturing of organoids along with immune cells has shown successive progress in creating better models and understanding the cancer progression in many research works. Though organoid technology also has various limitations various methods have been established to overcome the limitations and hence organoids can be used as an effective tool in cancer research and cancer treatment.

Acknowledgements

We would like to thank Ms. Amudha Madhavan for her critical review and proof reading of the chapter.

Acronyms and abbreviations

GEMMs	Genetically Engineered Mouse Models
PDTXs	Patient-derived xenografts
PDTOs	patient-derived organoids
iPSCs	pluripotent stem cells
human Pluripotent Stem Cells	hPSCs
Adult Stem Cells	ASCs

Author details

Allen Thayakumar Basanthakumar[1*], Janitha Chandrasekhar Darlybai [2] and Jyothsna Ganesh[2]

1 Dana Farber Cancer Institute, Boston, MA, USA

2 Mitra Biotech, Woburn, MA, USA

*Address all correspondence to: allenthayakumar@gmail.com

References

[1] Stratton MR, Campbell PJ, Futreal PA. The cancer genome. Nature. 2009;**458**(7239):719-724

[2] Luch A. Nature and nurture-lessons from chemical carcinogenesis. Nature Reviews. Cancer. 2005;**5**(2):113-125

[3] Radhakrishnan P, Baraneedharan U, Veluchamy S, Dhandapani M, Pinto DD, Thiyagarajan S, et al. Inhibition of rapamycin-induced AKT activation elicits differential antitumor response in head and neck cancers. Cancer Research. 2013;**73**(3 :1118-1127

[4] Starlin T, Saravana Prabha P, Allen Thayakumar B, Gopalakrishnan VK. Screening and GC-MS profiling of ethanolic extract of Tylophora pauciflora. Bioinformation. 2019;**15**(6):425-429

[5] Smalley M, Natarajan S, Mondal J, Best D, Goldman D, Shanthappa B, Pellowe M, et al. Nanoengineered disruption of heat shock protein 90 targets drug-induced resistance and relieves natural killer cell suppression in breast cancer. Cancer Research. 2020;**80**(23):5355-5366

[6] Ikpeazu C, Smalley M, Ulaganathan B, Thayakumar A, Majeiko L, Ganesh J, et al. Abstract LB-346: Case study: Non-uniform response to therapy in multiple metastatic is predicted using CANscript, a live tissue, ex-vivo, platform. AACR Annual Meeting. 2018;**78**:(13). DOI: 10.1158/1538-7445.AM2018-LB-346

[7] Ikpeazua C, Smalley M, Ulaganathan B, Thayakumar A, Basavaraja S, Gertje H, et al. Profiling metastatic lesions from a pembro-refractory patient to reveal distinct genomic instabilities and non-uniform response to drug combinations, ex vivo. Journal of Clinical Oncology. 2018;**36**:15

[8] Smalley M, Shanthappa BU, Gertje H, Lawson M, Ulaganathan B, Thayakumar A, et al. Therapy-induced priming of natural killer cells predicts patient-specific tumor rejection in multiple breast cancer indications. SABCS. 2017;**630**

[9] Smalleyc M, Shanthappa BU, Gertje H, Lawson M, Ulaganathan B, Thayakumar A, et al. Characterizing immunotherapy-induced lymphocyte infiltration at the single patient level using CANscriptTM, an ex-vivo human tumor model. Immunotherapy of cancer. 2017;**5**

[10] Corro C, Novellasdemunt L, Li XVSW. A brief history of organoids. American Journal of Physiology. Cell Physiology. 2020;**319**:C151-C165

[11] Drost J, Clevers H. Organoids in cancer research. Nature Reviews. Cancer. 2018;**18**(7):407-418

[12] McGranahan N, Swanton C. Clonal heterogeneity and tumor evolution: Past, present, and the future. Cell. 2017;**168**(4):613-628

[13] Bleijs M, van deWeteringM, Clevers H, Drost J. Xenograft and organoid model systems in cancer research. The EMBO Journal. 2019;**38**(15):e101654

[14] Sundaram M, Ulaganathan B, Dhandapani M, Thayakumar A, Mukhopadhyay P, Thiyagarajan S, et al. Abstract 3736: Application of patient tumors-derived tumor ecosystem platform for the development of novel

HDAC inhibitor in solid cancers. AACR Annual Meeting. 2014;**74**

[15] Fan H, Demirci U, Chen P. Emerging organoid models: Leaping forward in cancer research. Journal of Hematology & Oncology. 2019;**12**:142

[16] Sachs N, de Ligt J, Kopper O, Gogola E, Bounova G, Weeber F, et al. A living biobank of breast cancer organoids captures disease heterogeneity. Cell. 2018;**172**(373-86):e10

[17] Boretto M, Maenhoudt N, Luo X, Hennes A, Boeckx B, Bui B, et al. Patient-derived organoids from endometrial disease capture clinical heterogeneity and are amenable to drug screening. Nature Cell Biology. 2019;**21**:1041-1051

[18] Driehuis E, Kretzschmar K, Clevers H. Establishment of patient-derived cancer organoids for drug screening applications. Nature Protocols. 2020;**15**(10):3380-3409

[19] Majumder B, Baraneedharan U, Thiyagarajan S, Radhakrishnan P, Narasimhan H, Dhandapani M, et al. Predicting clinical response to anticancer drugs using an *ex vivo* platform that captures tumour heterogeneity. Nature Communications. 2015;**6**:6169

[20] Holloway EM, Capeling MM, Spence JR. Biologically inspired approaches to enhance human organoid complexity. Development. 2019;**146**(8):dev166173

[21] Junttila MR, de Sauvage FJ. Influence of tumour microenvironment heterogeneity on therapeutic response. Nature. 2013;**501**:346-354

[22] Sachs N, Clevers H. Organoid cultures for the analysis of cancer phenotypes. Current Opinion in Genetics & Development. 2014;**24**:68-73

[23] Shroyer NF. Tumor organoids fill the niche. Cell Stem Cell. 2016;**18**(6):686-687

[24] Fatehullah A, Tan SH, Barker N. Organoids as an in vitro model of human development and disease. Nature Cell Biology. 2016;**18**(3):246

[25] Onuma K, Ochiai M, Orihashi K, Takahashi M, Imai T, Nakagama H, et al. Genetic reconstitution of tumorigenesis in primary intestinal cells. Proceedings of the National Academy of Sciences. 2013;**110**(27):11127-11132

[26] Broutier L, Mastrogiovanni G, Verstegen MM, Francies HE, Gavarro LM, Bradshaw CR, et al. Human primary liver cancer–derived organoid cultures for disease modeling and drug screening. Nature Medicine. 2017;**23**(12):1424

[27] Sato T, Clevers H. SnapShot: Growing organoids from stem cells. Cell. 2015;**161**:1700-1700.e1

[28] Sato T, Stange DE, Ferrante M, Vries RG, Van Es JH, Van den Brink S, et al. Long-term expansion of epithelial organoids from human colon, adenoma, adenocarcinoma, and Barrett's epithelium. Gastroenterology. 2011;**141**:1762-1772

[29] Sato T, Clevers H. Growing self-organizing mini-guts from a single intestinal stem cell: Mechanism and applications. Science. 2013;**340**:1190-1194

[30] Sebert M, Denadai-Souza A, Quaranta M, Racaud-Sultan C, Chabot S, Lluel P, et al. Thrombin modifies growth, proliferation and apoptosis of human colon organoids: A protease-activated receptor 1- and protease-activated

receptor 4-dependent mechanism. British Journal of Pharmacology. 2018;**175**:3656-3668

[31] Kerr-Conte J, Pattou F, Lecomte-Houcke M, Xia Y, Boilly B, Proye C, et al. Ductal cyst formation in collagen-embedded adult human islet preparations. A means to the reproduction of nesidioblastosis in vitro. Diabetes. 1996;**45**(8):1108-1114

[32] Lee J, Sugiyama T, Liu Y, Wang J, Gu X, Lei J, et al. Expansion and conversion of human pancreatic ductal cells into insulin-secreting endocrine cells. eLife. 2013;**2**:e00940

[33] Turco MY, Gardner L, Hughes J, Cindrova-Davies T, Gomez MJ, Farrell L, et al. Long-term, hormone-responsive organoid cultures of human endometrium in a chemically defined medium. Nature Cell Biology. 2017;**19**:568

[34] Boretto M, Cox B, Noben M, Hendriks N, Fassbender A, Roose H, et al. Development of organoids from mouse and human endometrium showing endometrial epithelium physiology and long-term expandability. Development. 2017;**144**:1775-1786

[35] Lancaster MA, Knoblich JA. Organogenesis in a dish: Modeling development and disease using organoid technologies. Science. 2014;**345**(6194):1247125

[36] Lee JH, Bhang DH, Beede A, Huang TL, Stripp BR, Bloch KD, et al. Lung stem cell differentiation in mice directed by endothelial cells via a BMP4-NFATc1-thrombospondin-1 axis. Cell. 2014;**156**(3):440-455

[37] Wilkinson DC, Alva-Ornelas JA, Sucre JMS, Vijayaraj P, Durra A, Richardson W, et al. Development of a three-dimensional bioengineering technology to generate lung tissue for personalized disease modeling. Stem Cells Translational Medicine. 2017;**6**(2):622-633

[38] McCauley KB, Hawkins F, Serra M, Thomas DC, Jacob A, Kotton DN. Efficient derivation of functional human airway epithelium from pluripotent stem cells via temporal regulation of Wnt signaling. Cell Stem Cell. 2017;**20**(6): 844-57. e6

[39] Koshiyama M, Matsumura N, Konishi I. Recent concepts of ovarian carcinogenesis: Type I and type II. BioMed Research International. 2014;**934261**

[40] Matano M, Date S, Shimokawa M, Takano A, Fujii M, Ohta Y, et al. Modeling colorectal cancer using CRISPR-Cas9–mediated engineering of human intestinal organoids. Nature Medicine. 2015;**21**(3):256

[41] Nakayama M, Sakai E, Echizen K, Yamada Y, Oshima H, Han T, et al. Intestinal cancer progression by mutant p53 through the acquisition of invasiveness associated with complex glandular formation. Oncogene. 2017;**36**(42):5885

[42] Schell MJ, Yang M, Teer JK, Lo FY, Madan A, Coppola D, et al. A multigene mutation classification of 468 colorectal cancers reveals a prognostic role for APC. Nature Communications. 2016;**7**:11743

[43] Gomez-Cuadrado L, Tracey N, Ma R, Qian B, Brunton VG. Mouse models of metastasis: Progress and prospects. Disease Models & Mechanisms. 2017;**10**(9):1061-1074

[44] Sachs N, de Ligt J, Kopper O, Gogola E, Bounova G, Weeber F, et al.

A living biobank of breast cancer organoids captures disease heterogeneity. Cell. 2018;**172**(1-2):373-386.e10

[45] Della Corte CM, Barra G, Ciaramella V, Di Liello R, Vicidomini G, Zappavigna S, et al. Antitumor activity of dual blockade of PD-L1 and MEK in NSCLC patients derived three-dimensional spheroid cultures. Journal of Experimental & Clinical Cancer Research. 2019;**38**(1):253

[46] Kopper O, de Witte CJ, Lohmussaar K, Valle-Inclan JE, Hami N, Kester L, et al. An organoid platform for ovarian cancer captures intra- and interpatient heterogeneity. Nature Medicine. 2019;**25**:838-849

[47] Lakhani SR. WHO Classification of Tumours of the Breast. 4th ed. Lyon: International Agency for Research on Cancer; 2012

[48] Lee GY, Kenny PA, Lee EH, Bissell MJ. Three-dimensional culture models of normal and malignant breast epithelial cells. Nature Methods. 2007;**4**:359-365

[49] Vining KH, Mooney DJ. Mechanical forces direct stem cell behavior in development and regeneration. Nature Reviews. Molecular Cell Biology. 2017;**18**:728-742

[50] Zhong X, Gutierrez C, Xue T, Hampton C, Vergara MN, Cao LH, et al. Generation of three-dimensional retinal tissue with functional photoreceptors from human iPSCs. Nature Communications. 2014;**2014**(5):4047

[51] Zhang Q, Schepis A, Huang H, Yang J, Ma W, Torra J, et al. Designing a green fluorogenic protease reporter by flipping a beta strand of GFP for imaging apoptosis in animals. Journal of the American Chemical Society. 2019;**141**:4526-4530

[52] Dunn KK, Palecek SP. Engineering scalable manufacturing of high-quality stem cell-derived cardiomyocytes for cardiac tissue repair. Frontiers in Medicine. 2018;**5**:1-18

[53] Adams JW, Cugola FR, Muotr AR. Brain organoids as tools for modeling human neurodevelopmental disorders. Physiology. 2019;**34**:365-375

[54] Ho BX, Qian Pek NM, Soh B-S. Disease modeling using 3D organoids derived from human induced pluripotent stem cells. International Journal of Molecular Sciences. 2018;**19**:936

[55] Nantasanti S, de Bruin A, Rothuizen J, Penning LC, Schotanus BA. Concise review: Organoids are a powerful tool for the study of liver disease and personalized treatment Design in Humans and Animals. Stem Cells Translational Medicine. 2016;**5**(3):325-330

[56] Zhou J, Su J, Fu X, Zheng L, Yin Z. Microfluidic device for primary tumor spheroid isolation. Experimental Hematology & Oncology. 2017;**6**:22

[57] Ben-David U, Ha G, Tseng YY, Greenwald NF, Oh C, Shih J, et al. Patient-derived xenografts undergo mouse-specific tumor evolution. Nature Genetics. 2017;**49**:1567-1575. DOI: 10.1038/ng.3967

[58] Vlachogiannis G, Hedayat S, Vatsiou A, Jamin Y, Fernandez-Mateos J, Khan K, et al. Patient-derived organoids model treatment response of metastatic gastrointestinal cancers. Science. 2018;**359**:920-926

[59] Seino T, Kawasaki S, Shimokawa M, Tamagawa H, Toshimitsu K, Fujii M, et al. Human pancreatic tumor organoids reveal loss of stem cell niche factor dependence during disease progression. Cell Stem Cell. 2018;**22**(3):454-67. e6

[60] Sato T, Vries RG, Snippert HJ, van de Wetering M, Barker N, Stange DE, et al. Single Lgr5 stem cells build crypt-villus structures in vitro without a mesenchymal niche. Nature. 2009;**459**(7244):262-265

[61] Ootani A, Li X, Sangiorgi E, Ho QT, Ueno H, Toda S, et al. Sustained in vitro intestinal epithelial culture within a Wnt dependent stem cell niche. Nature Medicine. 2009;**15**(6):701-706

[62] Serra D, Mayr U, Boni A, Lukonin I, Rempfler M, Challet Meylan L, et al. Self-organization and symmetry breaking in intestinal organoid development. Nature. 2019;**569**(7754):66-72

[63] Smalleyd M, Shanthappa B, Gertje H, Lawson M, Ulaganathan B, Thayakumar A, et al. Nonuniform T-cell infiltration induced by PD-1 checkpoint blockade, ex vivo, predicts distinct clinical response. Cancer Research. 2018;**13**:78

[64] Orkin RW, Gehron P, McGoodwin EB, Martin GR, Valentine T, Swarm RA. Murine tumor producing a matrix of basement membrane. The Journal of Experimental Medicine. 1977;**145**:204-220

[65] Turner DA, Baillie-Johnson P, Martinez AA. Organoids and the genetically encoded self-assembly of embryonic stem cells. BioEssays. 2016;**38**:181-191

[66] Wilson HV. A new method by which sponges may be artificially reared. Science. 1907;**25**:912-915

[67] Holtfreter J. Experimental studies on the development of the pronephros. Revue Canadienne de Biologie. 1944;**3**:220-250

[68] Weiss P, Taylor AC. Reconstitution of complete organs from single-cell suspensions of chick embryos in advanced stages of differentiation. Proceedings National Academic Science USA. 1960;**46**:1177-1185

[69] Steinberg MS. The problem of adhesive selectivity in cellular interactions. In: Locke M, editor. Cellular Membranes in Development. New York and London: Academic Press; 1964

[70] Yu J, Vodyanik MA, Smuga-Otto K, Antosiewicz-Bourget J, Frane JL, Tian S, et al. Induced pluripotent stem cell lines derived from human somatic cells. Science. 2007;**318**:1917-1920

[71] Radhakrishnan P, Goldman A, Ulaganathan B, Kumar AT, Maciejko L, Gertje H, et al. Predicting tumor-immune response to checkpoint inhibitors using a novel patient-derived live tumor explant model. Journal of Clinical Oncology. 2017;**35**(15_suppl):e20035-e20035

[72] Simian M, Bissell MJ. Organoids: A historical perspective of thinking in three dimensions. The Journal of Cell Biology. 2017;**216**(1):31-40

[73] Scanu T, Spaapen RM, Bakker JM, Pratap CB, Wu LE, Hofland I, et al. Salmonella manipulation of host signaling pathways provokes cellular transformation associated with gallbladder carcinoma. Cell Host & Microbe. 2015;**17**:763-774

[74] Yin Y, Bijvelds M, Dang W, Xu L, van der Eijk AA, Knipping K, et al. Modeling rotavirus infection and antiviral therapy using primary intestinal organoids. Antiviral Research. 2015;**123**:120-131

[75] Roerink SF, Sasaki N, Lee-Six H, Young MD, Alexandrov LB, Behjati S, et al. Intra-tumour diversification in colorectal cancer at the single-cell level. Nature. 2018;**556**:457-462

[76] Xu H, Lyu X, Yi M, Zhao W, Song Y, Wu K. Organoid technology and applications in cancer research. Journal of Hematology & Oncology. 2018;**11**:116

[77] Abbasi J. Patient-derived organoids predict cancer treatment response. Journal of the American Medical Association. 2018;**319**:1427

[78] Viardot A, Bargou R. Bispecific antibodies in haematological malignancies. Cancer Treatment Reviews. 2018;**65**:87-95

[79] Jacob F, Salinas RD, Zhang DY, Nguyen PTT, Schnoll JG, Wong SZH, et al. A patient derived glioblastoma organoid model and biobank recapitulates inter- and intratumoral heterogeneity. Cell. 2020;**180**(1):188-204

[80] Smalleye M, Alam N, Murmu N, Somashekhar SP, Ulaganathan B, Thayakumar A, et al. A live tissue platform allows dynamic measurement of neovascularization and prediction of clinical response in human breast cancer samples, ex vivo. SABCS. 2018

[81] Sundarama M, Thiyagarajan S, Dhandapani M, Brijwani N, Prasath A, Thayakumar A, et al. Human tumor derived Oncoprint® platform predicts molecular mechanism of sensitivity and resistance to Fragmin in pancreatic cancer. Cancer Research. 2013;**8**:73

[82] Majumder B, Ulaganathan B, Thayakumar A, Thiyagarajan S, Brijiwani N, Tewari B, et al. Abstract 1304: Identification of responders for Anti-CTLA4 in refractory colorectal cancers using CANScript™ platform. AACR 106th Annual Meeting. 2015;**75**

[83] Radhakrishnana P, Dhandapani M, Ulaganathan B, Thayakumar A, Thiyagarajan S, Pinto D, et al. Majumde P K. PAT-1102, a novel HDAC inhibitor exhibits potent anti-tumor efficacy in patient-derived refractory solid tumors. Cancer Research. 2013;**73**:8

[84] Rios AC, Clevers H. Imaging organoids: A bright future ahead. Nature Methods. 2018;**15**(1):24-26

[85] Kit-Yi Yam A. 3D Perspective on Human Organoids: Promising Models for Studying Brain Development and Disease. Life canvas technologies; 2020

[86] Garcez PP, Loiola EC, Madeiro da Costa R, Higa LM, Trindade P, Delvecchio R, et al. Zika virus impairs growth in human neurospheres and brain organoids. Science. 2016;**352**:816-818

[87] Jinek M, Chylinski K, Fonfara I, Hauer M, Doudna JA, Charpentier E. A programmable dual-RNA-guided DNA endonuclease in adaptive bacterial immunity. Science. 2012;**337**:816-821

[88] Tetteh PW, Basak O, Farin HF, Wiebrands K, Kretzschmar K, Begthel H, et al. Replacement of lost Lgr5-positive stem cells through plasticity of their enterocyte-lineage daughters. Cell Stem Cell. 2016;**18**:203-213

[89] Basak O, Beumer J, Wiebrands K, Seno H, van Oudenaarden A, Clevers H. Induced quiescence of Lgr5+ stem cells in intestinal organoids enables differentiation of hormone-producing enteroendocrine cells. Cell Stem Cell. 2017;**20**:177-190 e4

[90] Richardson DS, Lichtman JW. SnapShot: Tissue clearing. Cell. 2017;**171**:496-496.e1

[91] Jamieson PR, Dekkers JF, Rios AC, Fu NY, Lindeman GJ amd Visvader JE. Derivation of a robust mouse mammary organoid system for studying tissue dynamics. Development. 2017;**144**(6):1065-1071

[92] Kim M, Mun H, Sung CO, Cho EJ, Jeon HJ, Chun SM, et al. Patient-derived lung cancer organoids as in vitro cancer models for therapeutic screening. Nature Communications. 2019;**10**(1):3991

[93] Barkauskas CE, Chung MI, Fioret B, Gao X, Katsura H, Hogan BL. Lung organoids: Current uses and future promise. Development. 2017;**144**(6):986-997

[94] Breslin S, O'Driscoll L. Three-dimensional cell culture: The missing link in drug discovery. Drug Discovery Today. 2013;**18**:240-249

[95] Pampaloni F, Reynaud EG, Stelzer EHK. The third dimension bridges the gap between cell culture and live tissue. Nature Reviews. Molecular Cell Biology. 2007;**8**:839-845

[96] Huh D, Hamilton GA, Ingber DE. From 3D cell culture to organs-on-chips. Trends in Cell Biology. 2011;**21**:745-754

[97] Yum K, Hong SG, Healy KE, Lee LP. Physiologically relevant organs on chips. Biotechnology Journal. 2014;**9**:16-27

[98] Renouf DJ, Velazquez-Martin JP, Simpson R, Siu LL, Bedard PL. Ocular toxicity of targeted therapies. Journal of Clinical Oncology. 2012;**30**:3277-3286

[99] Zhong X, Gutierrez C, Xue T, et al. Generation of three-dimensional retinal tissue with functional photoreceptors from human iPSCs. Nature Communications. 2014;**5**:4047

[100] Dutta D, Heo I, Clevers H. Disease modeling in stem cell-derived 3D organoid systems. Trends in Molecular Medicine. 2017;**23**:393

[101] Bhatia SN, Ingber DE. Microfluidic organs-on-chips. Nature Biotechnology. 2014;**32**:760

[102] Wang Y, Wang L, Zhu Y, Qin J. Human brain organoid-on-a-chip to model prenatal nicotine exposure. Lab on a Chip. 2018;**18**:851-860

[103] Munsie M, Hyun I, Sugarman J. Ethical issues in human organoid and gastruloid research. Development. 2017;**144**:942-945

[104] Tekin H, Simmons S, Cummings B, Gao L, Adiconis X, Hession C. C, Ghoshal A, Dionne D, Choudhury S. R, Yesilyurt V et al. Effects of 3D culturing conditions on the transcriptomic profile of stem-cell-derived neurons. Nature Biomedical Engineering. 2018:1-15

[105] Lukonin I, Zinner M, Liberali P. Organoids in image-based phenotypic chemical screens. Experimental & Molecular Medicine. 2021;**53**:1495-1502

[106] Drost J, van Jaarsveld RH, Ponsioen B, Zimberlin C, van Boxtel R, Buijs A, et al. Sequential cancer mutations in cultured human intestinal stem cells. Nature. 2015;**521**(7550): 43-47

[107] Yao Y, Xu X, Yang L, Zhu J, Wan J, Shen L, et al. Patient-derived organoids predict chemoradiation responses of locally advanced rectal cancer. Cell Stem Cell. 2020;**26**(1):17-26

[108] Ooft SN, Weeber F, Dijkstra K, McLean CM, Kaing S, Vanwerkhoven E, et al. Patient-derived organoids can predict response to chemotherapy in metastatic colorectal cancer patients. Science Translational Medicine. 2019;**11**(513):eaay2574

[109] Jabs J, Zickgraf FM, Park J, Wagner S, Jiang X, Jechow K, et al. Screening drug effects in patient-derived cancer cells links organoid responses to genome alterations. Molecular Systems Biology. 2017;**13**:955

[110] Workman MJ, Mahe MM, Trisno S, Poling HM, Watson CL, Sundaram N, et al. Engineered human pluripotent-stem-cell-derived intestinal tissues with a functional enteric nervous system. Nature Medicine. 2017;**23**:49-59

[111] Boussaad I, Cruciani G, Bolognin S, Antony P, Dording CM, Kwon YJ, et al. Integrated, automated maintenance, expansion and differentiation of 2D and 3D patient-derived cellular models for high throughput drug screening. Scientific Reports. 2021;**11**:439

[112] Kasendra M, Tovaglieri A, Sontheimer-Phelps A, Jalili-Firoozinezhad S, Bein A, Chalkiadaki A, et al. Development of a primary human small intestine-on-a-Chip using biopsy-derived organoids. Scientific Reports. 2018;**8**:287

[113] Dayem AA, Lee SB, Kim K, Lim KM, Jeon TI, Cho SG. Recent advances in organoid culture for insulin production and diabetes therapy: Methods and challenges. BMB Reports. 2019;**52**(5):295-303

Section 5

Organoid and Commercialization

Chapter 6

Organoids and Commercialization

Anubhab Mukherjee, Aprajita Sinha, Maheshree Maibam, Bharti Bisht and Manash K. Paul

Abstract

Organoids are 3D miniature tissue mimics and have been effectively used for various purposes, including disease modeling, various drug screening, mechanism of pathogenesis, stem cell research, and tumor immunology. Organoids are as varied as the body's tissues and organs and have enormous economic potential. They can open new ways to tailored therapy and precision medicine. In clinical investigations, patient-derived organoids have been used to predict patient responses to therapeutic regimens and perhaps improve cancer treatment outcomes. Recent developments in stem cell research and genomic technologies have led to breakthrough innovations in organoid bioengineering, large-scale manufacturing, biobanking, and commercialization. This chapter reviews the notion of organoid biobanking, companies involved and the commercialization aspect, and ethical considerations.

Keywords: organoid, tumoroids, commercialization, biobank, cell atlas

1. Introduction

Organoids are miniature 3D models of *in vivo* tissues and organs and faithfully mimic their structures and functions. These in vitro near-physiological models provide unique opportunities for diverse basic and translational human research applications [1]. Adult stem/progenitor cells from normal or diseased tissues are extracted for organoid creation. Guided differentiation of induced pluripotent stem cells (iPSCs), embryonic stem cells, and adult stem cells is followed by 3D culture on extracellular matrix using an appropriate culture medium to initiate organoid culture [2]. Long-term preservation of cells and organoids in biobanks is critical for future disease modeling, therapeutic development, regenerative medicine, toxicological studies, preclinical and personalized medicine (**Figure 1**). It is now possible to create organoids from various human tissues, including the airway, lungs, heart, brain, liver, brain, breast, gut, pancreas, and kidney (**Figure 2**) [3]. Another significant development is in the area of tumor organoids, which has opened up new avenues for human-specific tumor investigations, preclinical tumor studies, translating cancer research from the bench to the bedside [4].

Backed by some significant observations in the proliferative nature of adult tissue stem cells in 2009, the cardinal notion enveloping organoid technology is that stem cells have ingrained potential to self-assemble into 3D constructs with similitude with human organs [5]. As time rolled on, the modus operandi has been implemented

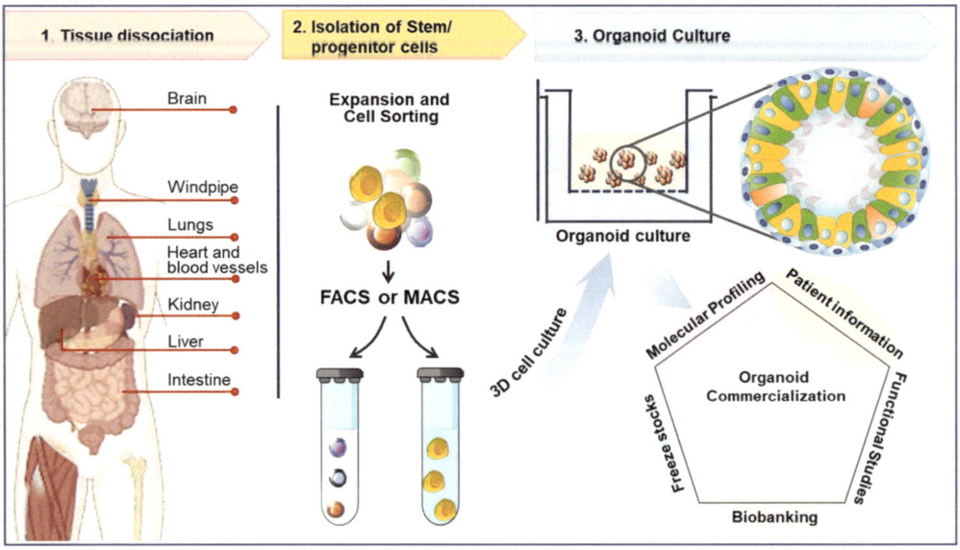

Figure 1.
Organoid formation from stem and progenitor cells. Following tissue dissociation, adult stem cell/ progenitor cells from normal or patients are isolated. Induced pluripotent stem cells (iPSCs), embryonic stem cells and adult stem cells are subjected to guided differentiation, followed by growing them on extracellular matrix in 3D culture system using specific culture media to begin organoid culture. The lower right section shows the different aspects of organoid commercialization, including molecular profiling of the collected cells, long term storage of cells with appropriate patient consent and information. These biobanked organoids can then be used for functional studies related to potential applications like disease modeling, therapeutic development, regenerative medicine, toxicology, and personalized medicine.

to produce several human and murine organoids out of epithelial tissues of various organs such as the liver, intestine, kidney, skin [6–9]. Another breakthrough entails the evolution of organoids obtained from induced pluripotent stem cells (iPSC), which can circumvent the toil to avail specific tissues like the heart or brain. This prodigious prospect, reinforced with genetic engineering, permits the mutational corrections in patient-derived iPSCs expediting differentiation to generate a specific type of cells [10–13]. Scrupulous experimental manipulation while maintaining sensitive biological complexity allows organoid technology to bridge the gap between 2D cell culture and 3D models [14]. It has also proved to better simulate human physiology than animal models and has shown the promise to substitute animals in preclinical biology [15, 16].

As ratiocinated from the trends, there will be a steady increase in the demand for organoid technology in the following years [3, 16]. As per reports published in various media, around 20 companies are into business with this technology—their activities include biobanking, manufacturing, commercialization, the implication of robotics for the development of organoids, organoids on a chip, etc. Statistically, priorities are given to heart, brain, intestine, and kidney organoids [3]. Financial models adopted by these companies are—(i) venture capitals, (ii) partnerships (iii) direct collaboration with the originators. Routine use of animals for disease modeling has always been afflicted with stringent moral and ethical queries. Usage of embryonic stem cells has also faced stormy skirmishes regarding the moral status of the embryos. Likewise, the moral and legal status of the organoids has been called in regulatory questions, to mention a few—ownership, consent, IP rights, safety, commercialization, etc.

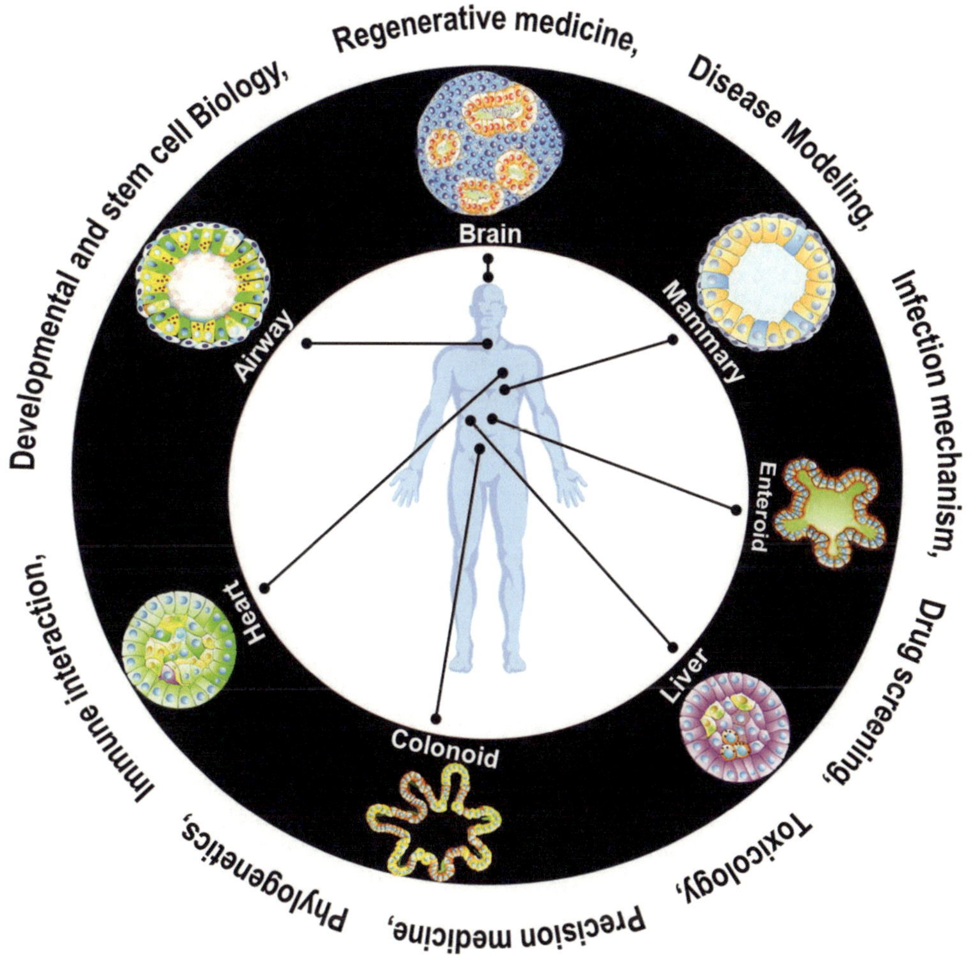

Figure 2.
Tissue specific organoid bioenginnering and different basic biomedical and commercial applications.

Utilization of 'matrigel' (extracellular matrix obtained from animals) has raised some safety concerns regarding compatibility with the human system. The debate revolving around the exchange or donation of human tissue as a commodity is still ongoing. To resolve this, few regulations should be declared and accepted by the global intellect [17]. Quibbles for intellectual property (IP) generation with human tissue should cease to persist, showing proper dignity and preserving the donor's rights. Consent should become a requirement avoiding de-identification of the donor [18–21]. In the present chapter, we shall highlight the usage of the organoid, organoid cell atlas, followed by shedding light on the commercialization aspect of the technology and future directionality.

2. Applications of organoids

Researchers traditionally used *in vivo* animal model systems and *in vitro* 2-D cell culture systems through decades for preclinical studies. Although these models have been demonstrated to be good and have provided invaluable insights into disease biology, they suffer from certain drawbacks. Excessive cell line passage introduces molecular and genetic alteration leading to variation from the original tissue phenotype and may not satisfactorily depict the original disease model's complexity and pathogenesis. The animal models may not appropriately reciprocate human disease development, suffers from ethical concerns, are very costly, and are time-consuming [17]. The recently developed 3D organoid technology, on the other hand, has evolved and opened up new options for basic and translational study and has fundamentally transformed *in vitro* disease research. Organoids can be easily manipulated, have the potential to recapitulate tissue complexity and physiology, and can be scaled up for high throughput drug screening because they have unique properties such as self-organization, lineage differentiation, signaling process, and maintenance of cell to cell communication, mimicking organ histology [17]. Human and animal cell-based organoid technology has advanced rapidly over the last decade [1], and various organoids mimicking several organs/tissues like the breasts [22], cerebral cortex [2], stomach, intestine [23], kidney [24], liver [25], lung [26–28], pituitary gland [29], prostate [30], pancreas have been developed.

With the advent of tumor organoid culture, patient-derived tumor organoids (PDTOs) have become popular tools to study molecular tumorigenesis, understand tumor heterogenity, predict drug responses, immunotherapy, and precision cancer therapy. At the moment, several tumor organoid biobanks have been developed catering to a variety of cancer types, including lung [31], breast [32], gut [33], and brain [34], liver [35], colorectal [36], pancreas [37], prostate [38], and ovary [39]. The role of tumor immune microenvironments (TIME) is significant in improving cancer immunotherapies, and PDTOs have started playing a crucial role in modeling the tumor-immune landscape. PDTO-based TIME studies can help evaluate immunotherapies such as checkpoint inhibition and adoptive T-cell treatment [4]. Thus, optimizing the tumor organoid culture method is critical for developing organoid-guided customized cancer immunotherapy [40].

Human organoids are suited for genetic modification and customization and bridge the gap between fundamental research and clinical practice. This technique has aided oncology, biological, pharmacological, regenerative, and personalized medicine studies [1]. Despite the initial advances, the technology is still nascent and is expected to be employed in various applications such as developmental and stem cell biology, toxicology, drug discovery, personalized medicine, disease modeling, immune interaction, and regenerative modeling (**Figure 2**). Healthy human organoids from different tissues may be utilized to test comparative therapeutic toxicities in combination with disease-related organoids. Cardiac organoids, liver organoids, kidney organoids, and other organoids are now used to dictate intolerable adverse effects, such as hepatotoxicity, cardiotoxicity, nephrotoxicity, and other tissue toxicity [41]. Patient-specific relevant organotypic models will go a long way in reframing basic findings, testing innovative ideas in 3D, and validating crucial data without sacrificing animal life for science. This aspect is dealt with in other publications [42, 43].

3. Application of tumor organoids

The lack of a physiologically relevant model system has delayed the therapeutic development process, and many candidates have failed in clinical trials [4]. Cancer organoids are near-physiological replicas of their parent tumors and bridge the gap between drug screening and clinical trials. Organoids have been utilized to examine personalized cancer patient responses in several research [32, 44, 45]. It may also be utilized to look at the epigenetic and genetic changes that cause drug resistance [46]. Tumor organoids can accurately predict chemotherapeutic response and resistance for certain drugs in some cancers [47, 48]. Finding the right therapeutic combination can be a challenge, and tumor organoids can help solve this dilemma and can make personalized medicine a reality [49]. The advances in genetic engineering technologies like CRISPR-Cas9 are implemented on organoids further to confirm medication sensitivity to specific mutations [50]. Organoids may also be used for pharmacokinetic research, critical in drug development. Results suggest that drug-transporters, their efflux transport functions, drug-metabolism can be efficiently studied using organoids [51]. In addition to cancer biobanks, organoids have a significant role to play in immunotherapy, a kind of cancer treatment in which the patient's immune system is used to eliminate tumor cells [52]. Organoid-based models are explored to study the effect of tumor-immune cell interaction using a coculture system with both components [53].

4. Organoid cell atlas

Organoids holds promise as a propitious platform in biomedical research and applications for many decades to come. Human organoids currently have a few limitations that require to be circumvented to appreciate their full potential. Some technical and conceptual limitations may be addressed using single-cell sequencing and spatial profiling. Single-cell transcriptome/ epigenome sequencing and spatial profiling can provide a thorough idea about the composition of cells and the state of cells present within the organoids, which may help develop organoids as futuristic models of human biology. In combination with the Human organoids and single-cell technology, a pilot project has been launched within the Human Cell Atlas (HCA) as a "Biological network" (https://www.humancellatlas.org/euh2020/) [54]. HCA is a revolutionary global collaborative initiative aiming at advancing biomedical research opportunities and therapy using single-cell technologies (https://hca-organoid.eu/). This pilot project, under HCA, focuses on the single-cell characterization of organoids and other complex *in vitro* systems. It has been established to foster the assembly, internal control, dissemination, utilization, and linking of such big human organoid-associated datasets [54–56].

It is one of the six pilot projects funded by the European Union (EU) Horizon 2020 Framework Programme, which will be helpful in developing the first version of the Organoid Cell Atlas, which may be used as a nucleus for a broader, collaborative, global initiative. The HCA-Organoid association has eight partner Institutions, including EMBL's European Bioinformatics Institute institutions having experts in organoid technology, single-cell profiling, advanced imaging, and bioinformatics from Austria, Germany, the Netherlands, and Switzerland, and received €5 million by EU funding, as a part of the European contribution to the HCA project. Currently, the project mainly focuses on generating single-cell transcriptome, epigenome maps, and detailed imaging data in a selection of human organoids. The initial objective of the funded project is to derive and characterize two organoids, colon and brain, from 100 whole-genome-sequence individuals each, to have a record of normal population variation and have a reference for disease-centric research [56].

The colon and brain organoids were one of the first organs to which organoids were demonstrated, so comparatively, more advanced protocols for the two are available with HCA [2, 23]. Apart from this, the colon organoids are derived from adult stem cells while the brain is from the iPSCs, thus spanning the two primary sources of organoid derivation. Both of them have primarily been used for disease-centric studies. If the single-cell characterization of these organoids is done for many individuals, this can help facilitate various biomedical applications. Beyond the initial target, most of the data information in the project is generalized in a way to be applicable to various other types of human organoids. The HCA has also spoken about the possibility that they can collaborate with other institutes for different projects, which can pursue systematic single-cell profiling in other types of human organoids, to explore the possibility of interrelation with the Organoid Cell Atlas [56].

The main aim of the EU H2020 HCA-Organoid project is to build an Organoid cell atlas portal that may be equipped with the computational infrastructure and a web-based front end that makes the data easily accessible and analyzed. Some of the organoid-specific features that have been focused on while developing an Organoid portal include the interactive exploration of human organoid data, data-driven selection of organoids for functional experiments, and comparison of disease-specific organoids against reference collections of normal organoids.

This portal also focuses on providing the data of the corresponding primary tissues available in the HCA and also will work on showing interactive mappings between single-cell profiles of human organoids. These may be achieved using the algorithms that enable cell-cell alignments between these datasets. This portal is supposed to facilitate the use of organoids in biomedical experiments and encourage the use of organoids as models in various experiments like precision medicine, drug development, disease modeling, etc. Mapping and data integration may detect normal variation between individuals in an interactive manner showcasing organoid as the capable model for the corresponding variation in primary tissues. The analysis and interpretations of disturbances in the human organoids related to the primary tissues will be performed using cell-cell alignments [56].

A set of strategies have been laid to develop the atlas to be most productive and of high quality. Initially, it was thought to invest in validation and standardization for organoid-related research. Later, a contribution towards the HCA to establish community standards and software infrastructure for data processing and data annotation was strategized. Then the development and validation of computational methods for the comparison of cells between organoids and corresponding primary tissues and their flexible alignments were implemented. Finally, the implementation of interactive visualization tools that helps in establishing user-friendly quality control and exploratory analysis of single-cell organoid datasets contributed to the Organoid Cell Atlas [55].

5. Commercialization of organoids

With the development and successful commercialization of organoids, the most demanded sector in treating patients and pre-clinical trials in pharmaceutical industries will give a slanting graph in the market in the future [57]. In this present era, many specific and most suitable techniques have been developing over the years for organoid research, leading to competition among industries worldwide. The annual cost of treating brain diseases in Europe is $798 billion, and globally it amounts to $3 trillion. Over 90% of novel drugs that are being developed for brain diseases fail during the developmental process, which further reinforces the scope and opportunities for organoids [2]. The development of the living human brain (LHB) enables culturing of human-derived brain organoids from the cells of any individual; the University of Helsinki provides a new technical idea for preclinical trials of drugs in this area. Helsinki Innovation Services Ltd (HIS) supports the commercialization projects of the University of Helsinki from the funding application stage to completion.

Many startups such as XILIS, CELLESCE, SYSTEM1 BIOSCIENCES, 3DYNAMICS, PATH BIOANALYTICS, KNOWN MEDICINE, CYPRE, DYNOMICS are currently working in the domain of organoid technology. XILIS is developing a patient-derived miniature organoid technology to upgrade precision medicine and pharmaceutical drug discovery; their needed materials lead to 30× speed, 50× throughput, and 300× cost-saving (Hans Clever includes in the founding team of XILIS). CELLESCE is a UK-based startup that invented a bio-processing technology intended to grow and expand organoids in drug discovery and regenerative medicine. $25 million of Series A venture funding is raised in SYSTEM1 BIOSCIENCES incorporation with Charles River Ventures and Pfizer Ventures, upgrading neuro drug discovery through the combined action of human brain models, scaled biology, and machine learning to interpret brain disease from genetics to neural computation. Also, KNOWN MEDICINE raised a total of $2.4 M from Khosla, Cota Capital, and Y-Combinator, offering cutting-edge biology research and the latest AI techniques, giving oncologists an easy spot for treating patient's tumors with the best suitable drug. PATH BIOANALYTICS does bioanalysis of Phenotypic drug discovery and development. CYPRE is developing a tumor model platform intended for transformative 3D cellular research and clinical testing of cancer patients with seed funding from Hemi Ventures and others. DYNOMICS received $500K in pre-seed funding from Boost VC. The details of the organoid-specific startups are presented in **Table 1**. These different startups contribute a vast platform to save millions of people's life [58]. Several companies are also operational in the tumor organoid domain, like Charles River and CROWNBio.

Company name	Country	Application area
XILIS INC.	Durham, North Carolina, USA	Micro-organospheres
CELLESCE	Wales, UK	Patient-derived organoids (PDO)
SYSTEM 1 BIOSCIENCES	San Francisco, CA, USA	Brain organoids
3DNAMICS	Baltimore, Maryland, USA	Brain and liver organoids
PATH BIOANALYTICS	North Carolina, USA	PDO for precision medicine
KNOWN MEDICINE	Salt Lake City, Utah, USA	Patient-specific organoids for cancer drug development
CYPRE	San Francisco, CA, USA	3D tumor model
DYNOMICS INC.	San Francisco, CA, USA	Human cardiac organoid
CHARLES RIVER	Wilmington, MA, USA	Tumor organoid
CROWNBio	San Diego, CA, USA	Tumor organoid

Table 1.
The current leaders in the commercialization of organoids, their geographical location, and application areas.

Despite using pre-clinical trials in animal models, concerns are raised about whether the animals will be extinct if used over the years. This will lead to the depletion of species and a significant effect on the ecosystem. Moreover, they may lead to harmful effects on the environment once mutated and released. The Animal Welfare Act of 1970 was implemented in the United States and set standards for animal use and care in research. Three principles of the Act are (1) experiments must be proven necessary for instruction or to save or prolong human life, (2) animals must be appropriately anesthetized, (3) animals must be killed as soon as the experiment is over. Much to our intrigue, different types of organoids such as kidney organoids, lung organoids, liver organoids, intestine organoids, brain organoids, etc., can substitute such animal models in preclinical trials for drug discovery and precision medicine. Even self-organ plantation may occur with the continuous development of organoids.

Globally, the expenses of organ transplantation and post-transplantation maintenance treatment are quite expensive but varies according to variables such as geographical location, medical facility, transplant organ type, and access to insurance coverage [59]. Private hospitals in India now charge around INR 10 lakh to INR 30 lakh for a heart transplant, while in USA, the charges can be very high ~$1,664,800.00 (https://www.statista.com/statistics/808471/organ-transplantation-costs-us/). While the cost of a kidney transplant goes from INR 5 lakh to INR 20 lakh, while in USA it can be around ~$442,500.00. The cost of a liver transplant runs from INR 15 lakh to INR 35 lakh, and ~$878,400.00 in the USA. The eventuality of the unaffordability of such expensive treatment modalities led to the demise of a multitude. Furthermore, organ transplants from other donors are sometimes associated with organ rejection and the onset of auto-immune disease. It is not only the high cost of transplant but also the availability and transport of organs is a major issue in many countries. Though the number of donors have increased but the needs have also reached new heights [59]. One-third of all organ transplants fail due to rejection due to multiple reasons including HLA mismatch and alloantibodies [60]. While modern medicine has halted acute rejection but chronic rejection is a major challenge. The organoid technology may provide a realistic patform to design transplantable tissues in a dish thereby catering to the transplant problem in the near future as current limitation prevent organoids from meeting these expectations.

Another recent scientific area where organoids showed great potential was during the COVID-19 pandemic caused by the SARS-CoV-2 coronavirus. SARS-CoV-2 causes respiratory illness and multi-organ dysfunction. Scientists were scrambling to test experimental COVID-19 systemic medicines. Organoids were used to study the adverse effects of SARS-CoV-2 infection on human tissues and for the investigation of prospective therapeutic approaches. With the recent work on mini lungs organoids, a few of the drugs stemmed from the infection of the organoid models, representing a handful of possible treatments for COVID-19 [26]. Scientists must still develop methods to produce more complicated systems, such immune cells and blood arteries, to fully harness the technology [26]. Scientists must also find a way to swiftly and inexpensively produce thousands of identical organoids. Bioprinting is a potential new fast prototyping method that prints cells and accompanying matrices in 3D. Organoid bioprinting uses hydrogel-based bioinks to deposit various cell types that stimulate physiological signaling and can help commercialize the platform faster [61].

According to a study published by Fior Markets, the global organoids, and spheroids market is predicted to increase from USD 502.92 million in 2019 to USD 2794.79 million in 2027, with a CAGR of 23.91% from 2020 to 2027 [57, 62]. Till now, 19 companies are having an interest in organoid commercialization. Some of them are Thermo Fisher Scientific (Waltham, MA, USA), Merck (Kenilworth, NJ, USA), Corning (Corning, NY, USA), STEMCELL Technologies (Vancouver, Canada), Lonza (Basel, Switzerland), Prellis Biologics (San Francisco, CA, USA), Amsbio (Abingdon, UK), Cellesce (Cardiff, UK), DefiniGEN (Cambridge, UK), OcellO B.V. (Leiden, Netherlands), HUB Organoid Technology (Utrecht, Netherlands), 3Dnamics Inc. (Baltimore, MD, USA), Organoid Therapeutics (Pittsburgh, PA, USA), InSphero (Schlieren, Switzerland), etc. Organome (Baltimore, USA) and HUB (Hubrecht Organoid Technology) are dedicated to organoid biobanking, and other companies aim at manufacturing, organoid marketing, other related technologies. SUN Biosciences (Lausanne, Switzerland) and System1 Biosciences (San Francisco, CA, USA) use robotic automation tools for organoid generation. The semi-automated process enabled researchers to make retinal organoid production and selection faster using the algorithm. The MIMETAS (Leiden, Netherlands)—the organ-on-a-chip company, offers the second-best cell-based model after humans, using human cells growing in three-dimensional structures called Mimetas'OrganoPlates (microfluidics-based culture plates allowing culturing and screening of a range of organ and tissue models), which are affordable and available for nonspecialized end-users. With a consumption market share of about 46% in 2019, North America is the most important consumer of organoids, with Europe in second place. Key manufacturers of the global organoids market are Thermo Fischer Scientific, Merck, and Corning. The top three players took up a market share of about 75% in 2019. Byers of the report can access verified and reliable market forecasts, including those for the overall size of the global organoids' market in terms of revenue. The Organoids' market is segmented into 3D Organoid Culture and Biochemical Cues. In the case of Organoids application, the leading players are Biopharmaceutical Companies, Contract Research Organizations, Academics, and Research Institutes. The regional analysis covers North America (USA, Canada, and Mexico), Europe (Germany, France, UK, Russia, and Italy), Asia-Pacific (China, Japan, Korea, India, and Southeast Asia), South America (Brazil, Argentina, Columbia, etc.), Middle East and Africa (Saudi Arabia, UAE, Egypt, Nigeria, and South Africa) and predicts an upsurge in the usage of organoid technology across the globe in future.

Organoid Biobank is like a commercial bank with a similar modus operandi. In organoid biobank, collected samples from different sources such as stem cells, primary tissues, and biopsies were made into organoids and stored. The organoid samples can be taken from a healthy individual and a patient. These stored organoids are ready to use for different purposes. Organoid biobanks manage the database of organoids and a registry with all the patient details. These stored organoids can be tracked and used for wireless phenotyping with the help of radio-frequency identification (RFID) ultracompact chips inserted within them. The organoid biobanks store and transport organoids using liquid nitrogen.

6. Regulatory guidelines in organoid research

The regulatory rules for organoid research use and commercialization are not very well laid in many countries and needs an update. The scientific, ethical, and regulatory problems related to organoid research are subject to extensive regulatory scrutiny and controlled partly by federal laws and state laws in the US and pertain to International laws in case of foreign collaborations. United States Department of Health and Human Services (HHS) and the Food and Drug

Administration (FDA) regulations are implemented in organoid research [63–65]. Organoid research is subject to the Institutional Review Board (IRB) approvals. Many institutions have Embryonic Stem Cell Research Oversight (ESCRO) or Stem Cell Research Oversight (SCRO) committees that oversee research utilizing human ESCs or iPSCs. These committees are outlined in the National Academies Guidelines for Human Embryonic Stem Cell Research and help evaluate the scientific and ethical aspects. The special committees assess the current state of research, weigh the advantages and hazards, address related ethical problems, including informed consent from the donor, and evaluate suitable supervision methods as per the federal guidelines [63].

While in Europe, organoids research must be approved by the Research Ethics Committee (REC) as per the guidelines laid down by the European Medicines Agency (EMA). Different European countries also have their individual regulatory agencies. In India, the regulatory board is the Institutional Committee for Stem Cell Research (IC-SCR). At the same time, in China, the measures for Ethical Review of Biomedical Research Involving Human Subjects and Ethical Guidelines for Human Embryonic Stem Cell Research, are used as guidelines [66]. The manufacturing process of organoids for commercial purpose must fulfill the same standards as other pharmaceutical drugs, following good manufacturing practices (GMP) [64, 65]. Additional hurdles exist at the convergence of organoid technology and commercial clinical use, global rules relating to the heterogeneity of approved quality standards, privacy laws and data protection, patent laws and identifying ownership. As a positive step in this direction, the International Society for Stem Cell Research (ISSCR) has set new stem cell research guidelines in 2021 [67–69]. It is expected that organoid-based biotechnology innovations would need updated global regulatory guidelines and governance in the future.

7. Ethics of organoid commercialization

Organoid technology and biobanking have grown in recent years, paralleling the expansion of stem cell and organoid research. However, ethical, moral, and legal existential questions persist. One crucial aspect is establishing globally recognized consent procedures for research and clinical organoid biobanking protocol. Also, the ethical and moral implications for clinicians while using organ mimics should be called into question. Patenting concerns are bound to arise when organoids are distributed over the world. Collaborations between the public and commercial sectors may lead to data exchange, entitlement sharing, etc. Confidentiality decorum and global patenting rules for organoid rights are therefore evolving. Even the iPSC-based organoids bring new concerns around permission, commercialization, ownership, IP rights, safety, and marketing [70]. The proliferation of big data, genomics, biobanking, and the globalization of the biotechnology sector has complicated the task of setting universal ethical standards. The primary ethical consideration about organoids is who owns them and whether small organ mimics (similar to organs) can be traded? With the advances in organoid technology, where do we draw lines to differentiate between organoids and tissues/organs? Sample de-identification, donor consenting, and licensing rights need to be better defined, especially concerning organoid commercialization. Addressing these bottlenecks may allow quicker commercial application for drug discovery, disease modeling, and research and development.

8. Conclusion

In the upcoming years, the designed pilot project focuses on substituting animal or human models with the organoid model by encouraging better research and accessibility of organoids. The HCA has been encouraging this shift of models by establishing a reference map of the entire human cells; which will be the first molecular picture of a human that will help the researchers to functionally dissect and systematically analyze human biological systems that would lead to a better exploration of organoids as a model. The initial version of the organoid cell atlas is planned to be established by the upcoming year that will be practically useful and open to advancements. These are thought to help maximize the impact of the project to become helpful in the field of basic biology and biomedical applications. To broader the reach, the single-cell profiles will be made public as soon as possible following HCA's ethical, social, and legal guidelines. Finally, the Organoid Cell Atlas Portal will be made "into a public, sustainable and widely used infrastructure for finding, accessing, analyzing and interpreting single-cell data from human organoids." The goal of the Organoid Cell Atlas is to make advancements in the biomedical field and develop various regenerative therapies by encouraging and accelerating disease-centric research of rare genetic diseases, precision oncology, or other complex diseases that are yet less understood. So, to achieve all of their objectives, they have made the portal open to create an inclusive research environment that would help in collaborating with a broad range of researchers interested in the field, which would later lead to extremely well-defined growth in the field of organoids.

Acknowledgements

M.K.P. acknowledges S. Dubinett, B. Gomperts, and V. Hartenstein for providing constant support and mentoring.

Conflict of interest

The authors declare no conflict of interest.

Author details

Anubhab Mukherjee[1], Aprajita Sinha[2], Maheshree Maibam[3], Bharti Bisht[4] and Manash K. Paul[5]*

1 Esperer Onco Nutrition Pvt. Ltd., Hyderabad, India

2 School of Biotechnology, Gautam Buddha University, Greater Noida, Uttar Pradesh, India

3 Department of Biochemistry, Manipur University, Imphal, Manipur, India

4 Department of Thoracic Surgery, David Geffen School of Medicine, University of California Los Angeles (UCLA), Los Angeles, CA, USA

5 Department of Pulmonary and Critical Care Medicine, David Geffen School of Medicine, University of California Los Angeles (UCLA), Los Angeles, CA, USA

*Address all correspondence to: manashp@ucla.edu; paul_cancerbiotech@yahoo.co.in

References

[1] Mahapatra C, Lee R, Paul MK. Emerging role and promise of nanomaterials in organoid research. Drug Discovery Today. 2022;**27**(3): 890-899

[2] Chhibber T, Bagchi S, Lahooti B, Verma A, Al-Ahmad A, Paul MK, et al. CNS organoids: An innovative tool for neurological disease modeling and drug neurotoxicity screening. Drug Discovery Today. 2020;**25**(2):456-465

[3] Takebe T, Wells JM, Helmrath MA, Zorn AM. Organoid center strategies for accelerating clinical translation. Cell Stem Cell. 2018;**22**(6):806-809

[4] Liu J, Huang X, Huang L, Huang J, Liang D, Liao L, et al. Organoid: Next-generation modeling of cancer research and drug development. Frontiers in Oncology. 2022;**11**

[5] Sato T, Vries RG, Snippert HJ, van de Wetering M, Barker N, Stange DE, et al. Single Lgr5 stem cells build crypt-villus structures in vitro without a mesenchymal niche. Nature. 2009; **459**(7244):262-265

[6] Lee J, Böscke R, Tang P-C, Hartman BH, Heller S, Koehler KR. Hair follicle development in mouse pluripotent stem cell-derived skin organoids. Cell Reports. 2018;**22**(1):242-254

[7] Huch M, Dorrell C, Boj SF, van Es JH, Li VSW, van de Wetering M, et al. In vitro expansion of single Lgr5+ liver stem cells induced by Wnt-driven regeneration. Nature. 2013;**494**(7436):247-250

[8] Takasato M, Er PX, Chiu HS, Maier B, Baillie GJ, Ferguson C, et al. Kidney organoids from human iPS cells contain multiple lineages and model human nephrogenesis. Nature. 2015;**526**(7574):564-568

[9] Sato T, Stange DE, Ferrante M, Vries RGJ, van Es JH, van den Brink S, et al. Long-term expansion of epithelial organoids from human colon, adenoma, adenocarcinoma, and Barrett's epithelium. Gastroenterology. 2011;**141**(5):1762-1772

[10] Spence JR, Mayhew CN, Rankin SA, Kuhar MF, Vallance JE, Tolle K, et al. Directed differentiation of human pluripotent stem cells into intestinal tissue in vitro. Nature. 2010;**470**(7332):105-109

[11] Lancaster MA, Renner M, Martin C-A, Wenzel D, Bicknell LS, Hurles ME, et al. Cerebral organoids model human brain development and microcephaly. Nature. 2013;**501**(7467):373-379

[12] Sanjurjo-Soriano C, Erkilic N, Baux D, Mamaeva D, Hamel CP, Meunier I, et al. Genome editing in patient iPSCs corrects the most prevalent USH2A mutations and reveals intriguing mutant mRNA expression profiles. Molecular Therapy - Methods & Clinical Development. 2020;**17**:156-173

[13] Mithal A, Capilla A, Heinze D, Berical A, Villacorta-Martin C, Vedaie M, et al. Generation of mesenchyme free intestinal organoids from human induced pluripotent stem cells. Nature Communications. 2020;**11**(1)

[14] Li M, Izpisua Belmonte JC. Organoids—preclinical models of human disease. New England Journal of Medicine. 2019;**380**(6):569-579

[15] Lancaster MA, Knoblich JA. Organogenesis in a dish: Modeling

development and disease using organoid technologies. Science. 2014;**345**(6194)

[16] Kaushik G, Ponnusamy MP, Batra SK. Concise review: Current status of three-dimensional organoids as preclinical models. Stem Cells. 2018;**36**(9):1329-1340

[17] Bredenoord AL, Clevers H, Knoblich JA. Human tissues in a dish: The research and ethical implications of organoid technology. Science. 2017;**355**(6322)

[18] Boers SN, Delden JJM, Clevers H, Bredenoord AL. Organoid biobanking: Identifying the ethics. EMBO Reports. 2016;**17**(7):938-941

[19] Perrone F, Zilbauer M. Biobanking of human gut organoids for translational research. Experimental & Molecular Medicine. 2021;**53**(10):1451-1458

[20] Mollaki V. Ethical challenges in organoid use. BioTech. 2021;**10**:3

[21] Mansour AA, Gonçalves JT, Bloyd CW, Li H, Fernandes S, Quang D, et al. An in vivo model of functional and vascularized human brain organoids. Nature Biotechnology. 2018;**36**(5):432-441

[22] Mohan SC, Lee T-Y, Giuliano AE, Cui X. Current status of breast organoid models. Frontiers in Bioengineering and Biotechnology. 2021;**9**:745943

[23] Sprangers J, Zaalberg IC, Maurice MM. Organoid-based modeling of intestinal development, regeneration, and repair. Cell Death & Differentiation. 2020;**28**(1):95-107

[24] Romero-Guevara R, Ioannides A, Xinaris C. Kidney organoids as disease models: Strengths, weaknesses and perspectives. Frontiers in Physiology. 2020;**11**

[25] Harrison SP, Baumgarten SF, Verma R, Lunov O, Dejneka A, Sullivan GJ. Liver organoids: Recent developments, limitations and potential. Frontiers in Medicine. 2021;**8**

[26] Sanyal R, Paul MK. Organoid Technology and the COVID Pandemic. SARS-CoV-2 Origin and COVID-19 Pandemic Across the Globe. IntechOpen; 24 June 2021. [Published]. DOI: 10.5772/intechopen.98542

[27] Paul Manash K, Bisht B, Darmawan Daphne O, Chiou R, Ha Vi L, Wallace William D, et al. Dynamic changes in intracellular ROS levels regulate airway basal stem cell homeostasis through Nrf2-dependent notch signaling. Cell Stem Cell. 2014;**15**(2):199-214

[28] Wilkinson DC, Alva-Ornelas JA, Sucre JMS, Vijayaraj P, Durra A, Richardson W, et al. Development of a three-dimensional bioengineering technology to generate lung tissue for personalized disease modeling. Stem Cells Translational Medicine. 2017;**6**(2):622-633

[29] Cox B, Laporte E, Vennekens A, Kobayashi H, Nys C, Van Zundert I, et al. Organoids from pituitary as a novel research model toward pituitary stem cell exploration. Journal of Endocrinology. 2019;**240**(2):287-308

[30] Elbadawy M, Abugomaa A, Yamawaki H, Usui T, Sasaki K. Development of prostate cancer organoid culture models in basic medicine and translational research. Cancers. 2020;**12**(4)

[31] Li YF, Gao Y, Liang BW, Cao XQ, Sun ZJ, Yu JH, et al. Patient-derived organoids of non-small cells lung cancer and their application for drug screening. Neoplasma. 2020;**67**(02):430-437

[32] Sachs N, de Ligt J, Kopper O, Gogola E, Bounova G, Weeber F, et al. A living biobank of breast cancer organoids captures disease heterogeneity. Cell. 2018;**172**(1-2):373-386.e1

[33] Yan HHN, Siu HC, Law S, Ho SL, Yue SSK, Tsui WY, et al. A comprehensive human gastric cancer organoid biobank captures tumor subtype heterogeneity and enables therapeutic screening. Cell Stem Cell. 2018;**23**(6):882-897.e11

[34] Jacob F, Salinas RD, Zhang DY, Nguyen PTT, Schnoll JG, Wong SZH, et al. A patient-derived glioblastoma organoid model and biobank recapitulates inter- and intra-tumoral heterogeneity. Cell. 2020;**180**(1):188-204. e22

[35] Broutier L, Mastrogiovanni G, Verstegen MMA, Francies HE, Gavarró LM, Bradshaw CR, et al. Human primary liver cancer–derived organoid cultures for disease modeling and drug screening. Nature Medicine. 2017;**23**(12):1424-1435

[36] van de Wetering M, Francies Hayley E, Francis Joshua M, Bounova G, Iorio F, Pronk A, et al. Prospective derivation of a living organoid biobank of colorectal cancer patients. Cell. 2015;**161**(4):933-945

[37] Driehuis E, van Hoeck A, Moore K, Kolders S, Francies HE, Gulersonmez MC, et al. Pancreatic cancer organoids recapitulate disease and allow personalized drug screening. Proceedings of the National Academy of Sciences. 2019;**116**(52):26580-26590

[38] Beshiri ML, Tice CM, Tran C, Nguyen HM, Sowalsky AG, Agarwal S, et al. A PDX/organoid biobank of advanced prostate cancers captures genomic and phenotypic heterogeneity for disease modeling and therapeutic screening. Clinical Cancer Research. 2018;**24**(17):4332-4345

[39] Kopper O, de Witte CJ, Lõhmussaar K, Valle-Inclan JE, Hami N, Kester L, et al. An organoid platform for ovarian cancer captures intra- and interpatient heterogeneity. Nature Medicine. 2019;**25**(5):838-849

[40] Neal JT, Li X, Zhu J, Giangarra V, Grzeskowiak CL, Ju J, et al. Organoid modeling of the tumor immune microenvironment. Cell. 2018;**175**(7):1972-1988.e16

[41] Matsui T, Shinozawa T. Human organoids for predictive toxicology research and drug development. Frontiers in Genetics. 2021;**12**

[42] Kim J, Koo B-K, Knoblich JA. Human organoids: Model systems for human biology and medicine. Nature Reviews Molecular Cell Biology. 2020;**21**(10):571-584

[43] Ashok A, Choudhury D, Fang Y, Hunziker W. Towards manufacturing of human organoids. Biotechnology Advances. 2020;**39**

[44] Seidlitz T, Merker SR, Rothe A, Zakrzewski F, von Neubeck C, Grützmann K, et al. Human gastric cancer modelling using organoids. Gut. 2019;**68**(2):207-217

[45] Zhou Z, Cong L, Cong X. Patient-derived organoids in precision medicine: Drug screening, organoid-on-a-chip and living organoid biobank. Frontiers in Oncology. 2021;**11**

[46] Lee SH, Hu W, Matulay JT, Silva MV, Owczarek TB, Kim K, et al. Tumor evolution and drug response in patient-derived organoid models of bladder cancer. Cell. 2018;**173**(2):515-528.e17

[47] Vlachogiannis G, Hedayat S, Vatsiou A, Jamin Y, Fernández-Mateos J, Khan K, et al. Patient-derived organoids model treatment response of metastatic gastrointestinal cancers. Science. 2018;**359**(6378):920-926

[48] Weber C. Organoids test drug response. Nature Cell Biology. 2018;**20**(6):634

[49] Verissimo CS, Overmeer RM, Ponsioen B, Drost J, Mertens S, Verlaan-Klink I, et al. Targeting mutant RAS in patient-derived colorectal cancer organoids by combinatorial drug screening. eLife. 2016;**5**

[50] Takeda H, Kataoka S, Nakayama M, Ali MAE, Oshima H, Yamamoto D, et al. CRISPR-Cas9–mediated gene knockout in intestinal tumor organoids provides functional validation for colorectal cancer driver genes. Proceedings of the National Academy of Sciences. 2019;**116**(31):15635-15644

[51] Onozato D, Yamashita M, Nakanishi A, Akagawa T, Kida Y, Ogawa I, et al. Generation of intestinal organoids suitable for pharmacokinetic studies from human induced pluripotent stem cells. Drug Metabolism and Disposition. 2018;**46**(11):1572-1580

[52] Qu J, Kalyani FS, Liu L, Cheng T, Chen L. Tumor organoids: Synergistic applications, current challenges, and future prospects in cancer therapy. Cancer Communications. 2021;**41**(12):1331-1353

[53] Fiorini E, Veghini L, Corbo V. Modeling cell communication in cancer with organoids: Making the complex simple. Frontiers in Cell and Developmental Biology. 2020;**8**

[54] Haniffa M, Taylor D, Linnarsson S, Aronow BJ, Bader GD, Barker RA, et al. A roadmap for the human developmental cell atlas. Nature. 2021;**597**(7875):196-205

[55] Bock C, Boutros M, Camp JG, Clarke L, Clevers H, Knoblich JA, et al. The organoid cell atlas. Nature Biotechnology. 2020;**39**(1):13-17

[56] Regev A, Teichmann SA, Lander ES, Amit I, Benoist C, Birney E, et al. The human cell atlas. eLife. 2017;**6**

[57] Choudhury D, Ashok A, Naing MW. Commercialization of organoids. Trends in Molecular Medicine. 2020;**26**(3):245-249

[58] Wang Z, He X, Qiao H, Chen P. Global trends of organoid and organ-on-a-chip in the past decade: A bibliometric and comparative study. Tissue Engineering Part A. 2020;**26**(11-12):656-671

[59] Lewis A, Koukoura A, Tsianos G-I, Gargavanis AA, Nielsen AA, Vassiliadis E. Organ donation in the US and Europe: The supply vs demand imbalance. Transplantation Reviews. 2021;**35**(2)

[60] Gu Y, Wong YH, Liew CW, Chan CEZ, Murali TM, Yap J, et al. Defining the structural basis for human alloantibody binding to human leukocyte antigen allele HLA-A*11:01. Nature Communications. 2019;**10**(1)

[61] Mahapatra C, Lee R, Paul MK. Emerging role and promise of nanomaterials in organoid research. Drug Discovery Today. 2022;**27**(3):890-899

[62] Lee S-J, Lee H-A. Trends in the development of human stem cell-based non-animal drug testing models. The Korean Journal of Physiology & Pharmacology. 2020;**24**(6):441-452

[63] The Emerging Field of Human Neural Organoids, Transplants, and Chimeras. 2021

[64] Vives J, Batlle-Morera L. The challenge of developing human 3D organoids into medicines. Stem Cell Research & Therapy. 2020;**11**(1)

[65] Lensink MA, Boers SN, Jongsma KR, Carter SE, van der Ent CK, Bredenoord AL. Organoids for personalized treatment of cystic fibrosis: Professional perspectives on the ethics and governance of organoid biobanking. Journal of Cystic Fibrosis. 2021;**20**(3):443-451

[66] Peng Y-J, Huang X, Zhou Q. Ethical and policy considerations for human embryo and stem cell research in China. Cell Stem Cell. 2020;**27**(4):511-514

[67] Hyun I, Clayton EW, Cong Y, Fujita M, Goldman SA, Hill LR, et al. ISSCR guidelines for the transfer of human pluripotent stem cells and their direct derivatives into animal hosts. Stem Cell Reports. 2021;**16**(6):1409-1415.

[68] Turner L. ISSCR's guidelines for stem cell research and clinical translation: Supporting development of safe and efficacious stem cell-based interventions. Stem Cell Reports. 2021;**16**(6):1394-1397

[69] Anthony E, Lovell-Badge R, Morrison SJ. New guidelines for stem cell and embryo research from the ISSCR. Cell Stem Cell. 2021;**28**(6):991-992

[70] Rachamalla H, Mukherjee A, K. Paul M. Nanotechnology application and intellectual property right prospects of mammalian cell culture. Cell Culture - Advanced Technology and Applications in Medical and Life Sciences. 2021. DOI: 10.5772/intechopen.99146